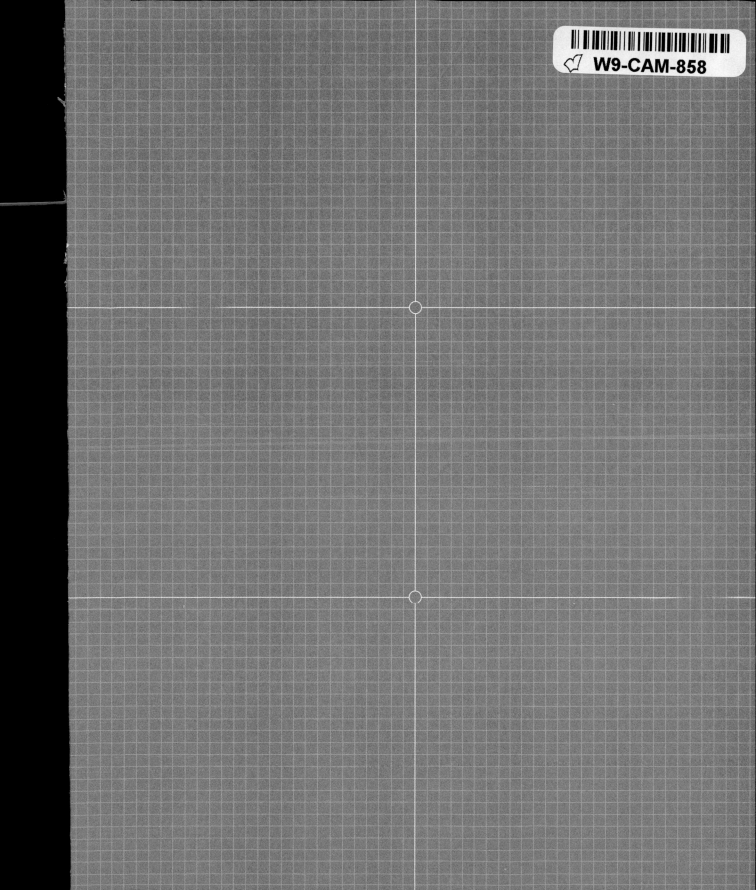

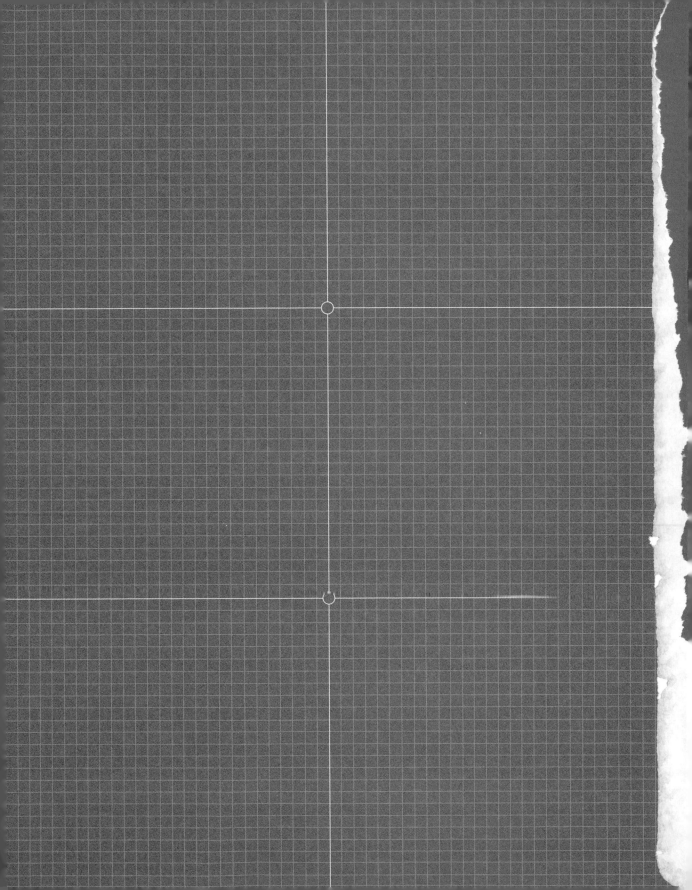

It's Not Just About Wrinkles

A Park Avenue Dermatologist's Program for
Beautiful Skin—in Just Four Minutes a Day

NEAL B. SCHULTZ, M.D., with Laura Morton

STEWART, TABORI & CHANG

NEW YORK

Editor: Jennifer Levesque
Designer: Nancy Leonard
Production Manager: Kim Tyner

Library of Congress Cataloging-in-Publication Data:

Schultz, Neal B.

It's not just about wrinkles : a Park Avenue dermatologist's program for beautiful skin
in just four minutes a day / by Neal B. Schultz with Laura Morton.

p. cm.

Includes bibliographical references and index.

ISBN 1-58479-407-0

1. Skin—Care and hygiene. 2. Beauty, Personal. I. Morton, Laura, 1964– II. Title.

RL87.S36 2006

616.5—dc22

2005032118

Photography credits: Pages 8 and 118: copyright © Francois Portmann; pages 10, 20, 21, 22, 23, 26, 27, 28, 29,
32, 53, 60 (bottom), 73, 75, 116, 162, 163, 168, 169, 172, 181, 182, and 187: copyright © Neal B. Schultz, M.D.;
pages 25, 34, 35, 47, 54, 58, 60 (top), 86, 110, 112, 153, and 173 copyright © Mitchell McCormack

Illustrations on pages 37, 159, 160, and 165: copyright © The Design Spot

Published in 2006 by Stewart, Tabori & Chang
An imprint of Harry N. Abrams, Inc.

The text of this book was composed in The Sans and Swiss

Printed and bound in Canada
10 9 8 7 6 5 4 3 2 1

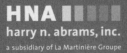

HNA

harry n. abrams, inc.
a subsidiary of La Martinière Groupe

115 West 18th Street
New York, NY 10011
www.hnabooks.com

DEDICATION

This book is dedicated to my patients, who have taught me the majority of what I know about the art of medicine; I will be eternally grateful for all they have given me. I have shared in their successes and failures, and our mutual respect has created a bond that makes my career far more rewarding than any other I can imagine. Their smiles and gratitude are priceless, and I am privileged to experience them every day.

CONTENTS

Introduction

FOR MORE THAN TWENTY-FIVE YEARS, I've enjoyed immense gratification in my career. In that time working as a board-certified cosmetic dermatologist on Park Avenue in New York, I've helped tens of thousands of patients improve the quality and appearance of their facial skin. The bottom-line result has always been a meaningful enhancement of my patients' self-esteem and overall sense of well-being—it's a no-brainer: when we look better we feel better. As a physician, it is truly rewarding to witness the newfound smiles of patients looking at their fresh reflection in the mirror. It's just plain fun to be able to share in the joy when my patients discover, with minimal effort, how to finally achieve the skin they've always wanted.

When it comes to your face, this book may be the most important resource you'll ever encounter. Like the Rosetta stone, it will be your ultimate guide in deciphering your skin problems. After reading this book, you

> *"Wherever the art
> of medicine is loved, there
> also is love of humanity."*
>
> **HIPPOCRATES**

---

will at last understand what your face needs, because I take the mystery, confusion, and complexity out of skin care by revealing dermatologists' trade secrets. This book will swing open the door to your having the flawless, younger-looking skin you've always wanted, but just didn't know how to get!

How? It's so simple.

Based on my clinically proven techniques, the book will not only help you identify what's really bothering you, but will also tell you how to fix it in simple-to-understand terms. You won't need a scientific or medical background to understand the techniques: You will learn how to identify what's really bothering you about your facial skin, including color issues such as red and brown spots and texture issues such as dry, flaky, dull-looking or large-pored skin. You will learn how to look into a mirror and identify your problem areas, by first learning what the problems are and why you have them. Most color and texture issues can be improved through my program. (More severe issues can be effectively dealt with by a qualified dermatologist, as discussed in chapter 13.)

You will also learn how to correctly identify your skin type, which is crucial to finding the right products to improve the quality and appearance of your skin. My program is predicated on knowing your correct skin type. Once you know your skin type, you will effectively learn to select the right products for your skin, which will help you recapture and restore your bright, radiant, youthful glow.

If you follow my four-step program for thirty days, you will see a noticeable difference in your complexion, with the improvement of any unwanted color problems and the presence of a softer, smoother texture.

By opening this book, you have entered a world previously unavailable to you. This world will help you repair and rejuvenate your skin, improve your complexion, and achieve

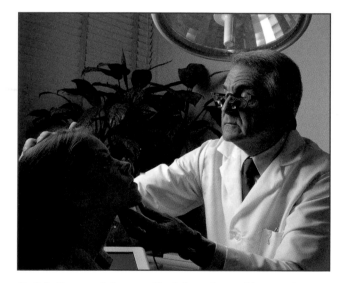

Dr. Schultz examining a patient for color and texture issues.

your desired results. That way, you can return to your everyday world with an empowering sense of confidence. And human nature drives us all to want to be better: better looking, *better feeling,* and just plain better in every way.

During almost three decades of practice, I have witnessed and treated every imaginable (and unimaginable) facial-skin problem out there. With my twelve thousand patients a year, I've seen it all, and I've dealt with each condition on a very personal level. So I know that, if you're like most of my patients, you simply don't accurately understand your skin flaws. My patients make it abundantly clear they have no idea what the issues are that constitute their skin problems in the first place. I'll hold a mirror in front of their face and ask them to point out what it is they don't like about the way they look, and most can tell me they want to look better and have a healthier, better-looking face. But they can't describe with any accuracy *specifically* what they don't like about their skin, with one exception: they can, of course, point out those darn wrinkles, since they are the easiest flaws to articulate—we all know what a wrinkle looks like!

Let's face it (sorry about the pun): We live in a monomaniacal world focused on lines and wrinkles, and most skin-care professionals are feeding right into it. But wrinkles are just a small part of the big picture, and that's why I've written this book—it's *not* just about wrinkles. To better understand what I mean, read on.

The biggest misconception in facial-skin care today is that lines and wrinkles are the only problems that cause you dissatisfaction with your skin. *Not true!* It is the *color and texture* issues that probably account for your disappointment. Ninety-five million women are affected by color and texture ailments, but only 42 million have lines and wrinkles. You will quickly learn that lines and wrinkles are actually the *least* important component of the beautiful skin you've always wanted—but didn't know how to get.

THE AIM OF *IT'S NOT JUST ABOUT WRINKLES*

The main goal of this book is to provide you with all of the information you need to *identify what's wrong with your skin, remedy those skin flaws, and maintain your newfound luster and clarity.*

Skin care is a fiercely personal and intimidating subject, but with the help of this book you can achieve all of this in a nonintimidating environment from the privacy of your own home. I want to enable you to tackle your skin while lounging on your sofa, lying in bed, or drinking your morning coffee, without a stranger in a white coat staring at you, making you feel more awkward or uncomfortable about your appearance than you already do. Think of me as your own personal embedded dermatologist; I have gone behind enemy lines, worked in the trenches, and seen firsthand every possible ailment when it comes to facial-skin care. And now you have me fighting at your side to help you achieve your goal of healthier, better-looking skin.

After reading this book, you will not only understand how to accurately identify your correct skin type, you will also have learned how to select the right products (there are five: a cleanser, a toner, an active ingredient, a sunscreen, and a moisturizer) for your skin type, so that you will successfully recapture and restore your bright, radiant, glowing skin. Any fear or intimidation you have about skin care will be completely alleviated once you understand the simplicity of my program.

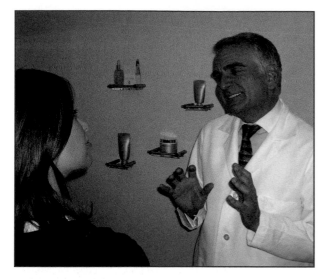

Dr. Schultz talking to a patient.

The entire world of skin care is really as easy as one, two, three:

1. Identifying your correct skin type
2. Determining your facial imperfections
3. Selecting and using the right products for you

How simple is that? Understanding these three easy steps will finally allow you to take control of your skin so that you can have beautiful skin forever.

So why has effective skin care been such a mystery until now? Because no one has ever explained it. No one has presented in layman's terms how you can identify what's *really* wrong with your skin when you look into a mirror. That is the first and most important step in winning the battle for younger, healthier-looking skin. For most people, skin care is a hit-or-miss proposition. In fact, most people don't even know their skin type (there are six), which is the most basic step in purchasing the correct skin-care products to remedy your ailments. Everything in this book is predicated on your skin type.

Before you can break out of your self-imposed prison, you must first realize you're locked up. Whatever you are trying to avoid about your skin won't go away until you confront it. This is the first skin-care book that allows you to learn about, understand, and then obtain treatment for your more important facial *color* and *texture* problems. Unlike skin-care books that are dedicated to the single defect of lines and wrinkles, my book addresses the *whole* picture of facial rejuvenation. The whole picture must include the more visibly important and compelling, but difficult to describe, subjects of texture and color. It is the *whole* picture that inspired me to write this book.

To me, wrinkles are just one of the moons of Jupiter in the universe of facial-skin defects; they are a very small part of what causes you to be discouraged or unhappy when you look in the mirror. Any woman who

ASK YOURSELF THE FOLLOWING QUESTIONS:

What do you want to change about your facial appearance? Can you identify color and texture issues? Why did you buy this book?

has put on makeup knows, without a doubt, that *it's not just about wrinkles.* As I said earlier, we live in a tunnel-visioned world that has put an emphasis on lines and wrinkles, and you are led to believe that when those lines and wrinkles are fixed, all of your facial imperfections will be cured. Sadly, that line of thinking misses the *whole* picture. In fact, for most of us, fixing lines and wrinkles is a minority factor in the overall quest for easily attainable beautiful skin. Look, if you have an old, rusted car with a dented door and you fix the dented door, you still have an old, rusted car! That's exactly the effect of the laser-like focus on fixing wrinkles: color and texture problems are ignored—problems we *all* have.

If you could change anything about your face, what would it be? When you look in the mirror, what do you see staring back? Your face is your ambassador to the rest of the world. Whether right or wrong, it's the feature other people use most in forming important first impressions. Take a few minutes and really examine your facial features with a hand mirror. First, use the nonmagnified side. Try to describe anything you'd like to see changed or improved. Chances are, you've easily identified your lines, or that w word, *wrinkles*. That's an easy start, but remember, wrinkles are a very small part of the *whole* picture in terms of improving your skin so you can smile when you look into any mirror.

Next, take a few minutes to examine your face again, but this time, use the magnifying side of the mirror. Yikes! It isn't what you were expecting, right? Now that you are seeing your face five times closer and the problems are five times more glaring, is there anything else that needs a "little fix"? I'll bet your answer is a resounding "*yes!*" As the old saying goes, "If you don't like what you see in the mirror, don't break the mirror, change the reflection." And that's why I'm here: I can and will help you do that. I hear your SOS—your plea for help—loud and clear, each and every day. I want to enable you to take control of your skin by revealing to you the "insiders' secrets" about how to restore, perfect, and then preserve your skin so that you can look and feel younger, and better, with a renewed sense of confidence and well-being. *Don't lie about your age . . . Let your skin do it for you!*

> **GET A TWO-SIDED MAGNIFYING MIRROR.**
>
> *Make sure you are sitting in a well-lit area. First, hold up the nonmagnifying side and examine your face. List the areas you think need improving, describing what it is that makes you think those areas are not right. Next, switch the mirror to the magnifying side (at least 5X). List all visible flaws you'd like to remedy.*

THE DISCONNECT

When it comes to skin-care products, manufacturers are doing the best they can to tell consumers what their products do. Unfortunately, it can be difficult for consumers to identify and recognize the different components of color and texture problems that the various skin products address. There are hundreds of products available, such as cleansers, toners, moisturizers, acne medications, alleged pore reducers, brown-spot faders—the list goes on and on. But when typical consumers look into the mirror, they can rarely determine which of those products will improve their color, texture, and contour problems. That's the quintessential *disconnect* between your unidentifiable facial-skin-care problems and the available, effective skin-care products out there.

Inevitably, every day in my office, when one patient sees another patient leaving with a product that she doesn't have, she immediately wants the other patient's product and wants to know why it was not included in her skin-care routine. It's the "I want what she's having" philosophy, even if what *she's* having isn't something *you* need. As is common, my patients want the newest, best, latest and greatest "product" in their quest to achieve perfect skin.

There is almost no relationship between the cost of a skin-care product and its effect. More expensive does *not* mean better. The reality is that most people buy the wrong products for their skin without any rational basis for buying them. The next time you buy a skin-care product, ask yourself the following questions: Why are you buying it? What do you want it to do for you? Each of us has individual problems and therefore needs a personalized program. What's good for your girlfriend's skin may not be right for yours. It's so important to personalize the selection of your skin-care products according to your own skin's problems and type. By addressing the *whole* picture, this book identifies the solution to *your* skin-care needs.

Every day, we are exposed to massive attempts at consumer marketing—which expands from person to person by word of mouth. And while that's great for my Web site, if you don't have the skills to sort through the advertisements and hearsay to help select the right products for your skin, you will never see the kind of improvement those products offer. Nothing can ruin the reputation of a product faster than word of mouth suggesting that it doesn't work, or even worse, that the product aggravates a problem. But, if you are putting the wrong fuel into the right vehicle, how can you expect it to perform to your expectations? *You can't fix a problem if you don't know what the problem is.* Understanding, integrating, and implementing the information in this book will enable you to finally target your individual needs.

IT'S *REALLY* NOT JUST ABOUT WRINKLES

I have patients who come into my office every day asking for Botox or fillers for their facial lines, because facial lines are the only element of their facial problems they can identify. Botox and collagen and other fillers can very effectively help lines and wrinkles, but they do nothing to solve color or texture complexion problems. Some of these patients do need their wrinkles fixed, while others have barely a visible line. Regardless, almost all of these patients have some kind of color or texture condition. I usually respond by saying, "I'll be glad to fix your wrinkles, but you still won't be pleased with your skin because it is not your wrinkles that are making you unhappy."

After I tell patients that Botox and fillers are not the answer and alone will not fix their facial problems, I hold a mirror up (like you just did) and show them the reds and browns in their skin. I demonstrate the places where their skin texture is dull—lifeless—and perhaps flaky. I point out any large pores and any place their makeup isn't adhering properly. As harsh as that seems, within sixty seconds they understand what I am saying. Yes, I can make those lines disappear—with ease. But I know if we don't take care of the other issues, my patients won't be completely satisfied.

The last thing I want is for patients to spend five hundred to a thousand dollars in my office, leave thinking they are going to be happy, and then discover it wasn't the lines they were dissatisfied with in the first place—it was their overall color, texture, and contour combination. Invariably, when I point out the larger issues, patients take my advice—and I end up with happy, more radiant, healthier-looking patients who are thrilled with the results. Their friends want to know their secret—and they tell them to "go see Dr. Schultz." That's the kind of word-of-mouth marketing every physician hopes for.

COLOR AND TEXTURE—AS PRECIOUS AS A DIAMOND

Ask any woman what type of diamond she'd like and she'll probably answer with the number of carats and her favorite shape. But what about color and clarity? These two elements are much more important when choosing a diamond. In fact, any jeweler will agree that of the four *c's*, color and clarity are far more meaningful in determining diamond quality than carat size or cut. If you want the best diamond, the one that sparkles and dances in every type of light, you want superior color and clarity—which are responsible for that perfect stone—not cut or carat size.

A comparison can be made when it comes to your facial skin. (And really, who wouldn't want their face to be likened to a diamond that sparkles in the light?) There are only three essential elements that determine, for better or worse, how your skin looks: *color, texture,* and *contour.* Every defect, dull spot, blotch, pimple, scar, pore, or mark—whether real or perceived—fits into one of these three categories. It's really that simple.

Color problems include red and brown spots, blotches, linear red marks, and discolorations. Some examples are freckles, caused by broken pigment (color) cells from the sun and aging, and broken capillaries, which are broken blood vessels (from female hormones, foods, alcoholic beverages, acne blemishes, and, of course, previous sun exposure).

Texture problems include dullness, flakes, scales, large pores, roughness, and cobblestoning. The reason your skin texture disappoints you and appears dull, matte, tired, and/or large pored is that there is an accumulation and piling up of dead cells both on the surface of your skin and inside your pores. This is the result of sun damage, aging (ugh!), and even genetics.

Finally, *contour* problems are the easiest to recognize. They most commonly consist of lines and wrinkles, but also include sagging skin, jowls, and under-eye bags. While these are certainly important issues, they pale in comparison to your skin's color and texture in contributing to the overall appearance of your skin.

Once you understand the simple components and the relationship of these three elements (and I will explain them in *simple and easy-to-understand terms* in chapter 1), you'll be able, at last, to identify imperfections in each of the three elements of your changing and aging skin. And because of this, you'll actually be able to find the correct skin-care products to fix your troubled skin.

What I've just described amounts to a skin-care epiphany, which represents my motivation in writing this book: someone finally needed to empower you, the consumer, with basic skin-care information for satisfactorily improving your complexion's overall appearance. After finishing this book, you will know, without any doubt, what your facial-skin problems are and how to select the right products for your skin. And you will realize you can do it without expensive prescription medications or visits to *my*—or any other dermatologist's—office!

SKIN IN HARMONY

Together, *color, texture,* and *contour* are to skin what musical instruments are to the orchestra. If skin color, texture, and contour are in balance, the appearance of your skin pleases your eyes, just as an orchestra's music pleases your ears when the instruments are properly tuned and in balance. The balance instills pride, happiness, and self-confidence. If these elements are out of balance, the visual cacophony can be the root cause of your unhappiness, frustration, and even shame. Unhappy skin makes for unhappy people.

If you follow my very simple program, which consists of understanding the three elements of your skin (color, texture, contour) and performing a personalized simple skin-care routine (which will only take you four minutes a day), you will see a rapid and noticeable improvement in your complexion's color and texture within the first fifteen to thirty days of your new skin-care routine. In fact, throughout this book you will see before-and-after photographs of real people who have been on my program with great success.

What we're talking about isn't a miracle. It's not even rocket science, but it *is* science. My sole purpose is to enable you to understand that the skin you want is well within your grasp. I don't need a high-profile celebrity to endorse my products or my professional techniques to establish credibility. I have a quarter of a century of experience and tens of thousands of happy and satisfied patients to do that for me. Everyday people—just like you. Once you get your skin's color and texture under control, you'll wear less (or even no) makeup—and any you do use will go on more smoothly and look better. That may seem totally out of your realm of possibility, but I have patients—stylish and meticulous Park and Fifth Avenue women—who hardly wear any makeup since learning the secrets and experiencing my skin-care techniques, home treatments, and products. And you want to know something? That's how *I* know I've succeeded. As a result, there are an enormous number of patients (women *and* men) who walk around looking better, feeling better, and showing the world what a difference education and the correct products make in reaching their skin-care goals.

Are you ready to become one of those people? I thought so—let's get started.

CHAPTER

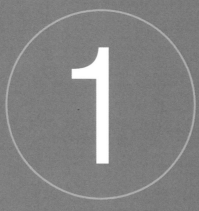

1

"The most beautiful thing we can experience is the mysterious."

ALBERT EINSTEIN

Color and Texture

I LOVE WHEN PATIENTS COME INTO MY OFFICE and say, "Doc, you think you could look at this thing?" and then point to a bump, an age spot, mild acne, or eczema. All of these ailments are simple color and texture issues that are easily treatable—if you know what you're treating—and in order to find out specifically what they are, patients have to feel comfortable enough with their dermatologist to talk about their symptoms. A recent study showed that most patients have only eighteen seconds to deliver their story before the doctor interrupts. But listening—and listening carefully—to my patients is how I figured out there was a real need for the information in this book!

The most important thing I learned in medical school—which I regret a lot of doctors don't understand—is that if doctors only listen to their patients, their patients will tell them what's wrong. Patients help with the diagnosis. Although most patients don't understand the nature of their problems, their words of frustration and unhappiness regarding their skin have been invaluable in empowering me to help them. Thankfully, that has helped me build a very strong practice and has offered me years of professional gratification. For years I've seen people with defects they thought they'd never be rid of blossom and flower as a result of their transformation. I get so much satisfaction from seeing people smiling and feeling better about the way they look. Self-perception is the reason you bought this book; it is the foundation for understanding the psychological bond we have to our overall appearance.

My approach to skin care involves what I call "the whole picture." I can fix wrinkles, but that won't address color or texture. I can pop a pimple, but that won't cure a chronic condition. If you were having a problem with the brakes on your car, you wouldn't ask the mechanic to make the horn louder, right? That's like a patient who comes in and asks for Botox for lines when what she really needs is a superficial peel or lasering for texture or color problems. She senses that something about the whole picture is off, but she is directed by our market-driven society to the wrong segment of the whole picture. Her response is partly psychological, but it's also influenced by the fact that her lines are the only skin defects that she can identify.

> **MORE THAN 3 MILLION**
>
> *workdays are lost each year because of skin diseases, with acne as the leading skin disease (occurring in 20 percent of all patients seeking treatment for skin disorders).*

I have a patient, a fifty-two-year-old woman, whose skin has rarely been exposed to the sun; her face is absolutely smooth, lustrous, and gorgeous. On top of that, she's had numerous cosmetic procedures. She's had her eyes done and her face lifted. She could easily pass for thirty-five. But she has a large, conspicuous mole right above her left eye—something she doesn't see when she looks into a mirror. As far as she is concerned, it's fine. Perhaps to some, that mole takes away from the beautiful skin she has worked so hard to achieve, but to my patient it's just a part of her—a part that she embraces. On the other end of the spectrum, there are women who will absolutely not tolerate a freckle or a broken capillary on their face, chest, or hands. My point is that *your* happiness is the ultimate goal in the pursuit of healthier-looking skin.

The skin is the body's largest and most visible organ. It reflects a person's general health and performs many important bodily functions. An average-sized person has twenty-one square feet of skin (about the size of some New York City apartments), which serves as the body's frontline defense against injury and infection. The skin also regulates body temperature, acts as a sensory and excretory organ, and synthesizes vitamin D when exposed to ultraviolet light. A vast network of blood vessels in the skin provides oxygen and nutrients to sensory and motor nerves, and also to all skin appendages, including oil and sweat glands, nails, and hair follicles. (For those of you who want to know more about skin's composition and function—you're my kind of people—see chapter 2.)

Not surprisingly, this complex, exposed organ is vulnerable to injury, disease, ailments, discolorations, and, of course, aging (sorry—don't blame the messenger). But you bought this book because you know you need help. You already know there's a problem that you can't seem to fix; maybe you've already been to a dermatologist and you've been unhappy with the results. Maybe you are too embarrassed to make an appointment. Whatever the case, I'm glad you're here to share in my treasure trove of practical knowledge.

Numerous types of marks and lesions can appear on the skin, especially as we grow older. (And by the way, it's OK to get older—we just don't want to get old.) Whether from the red of a pimple, or from the pink spots that turn into dark spots whenever the skin is injured, color issues appear on every face. But your color and texture issues started in your teenage years. Maybe it was that self-inflicted extrication of a zit (done with little grace or facility) that created a significant amount of damage to the upper levels of the skin, darkening the area and even creating a hole where the pimple was. Careless zit popping from teenage years can become a persistent color and contour problem later on. But it was easy, then, not to think of these issues; with the exception of pockmarks caused by chicken pox or scars from traumatic lacerations, contour issues are not a problem for most teens.

COLOR

Skin discoloration can be divided into two different groups: browns and reds. You might notice some blue hues, especially under and above the eyes and sometimes on the cheeks, but those veins appear blue for the same reason the sky is blue. It's called the Tyndall effect, and it's caused by the way light is scattered as it passes through objects. The blood those veins carry is only a little bit darker than the bright red blood in the deeper hidden arteries, but the Tyndall effect makes it look blue. So, for all intents and purposes, all color issues are defined by either brown or red.

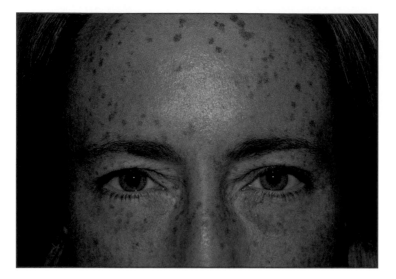

ABOVE AND BELOW: *Sunspots, age spots, and liver spots are all the same thing and can easily be removed.*

Browns

Whether sunspots, freckles, or brown patches of skin, browns are either diffuse or discreet. Brown spots appear in exposed areas including the face, back of the hands, chest, back, arms, and legs. The brown family runs a full spectrum of hues from light tan through medium and darker tan to lighter, medium, and darker brown. The principal cause of this type of discoloration is accumulated sun exposure, which causes the pigment cells (the cells that make our normal color) to produce more color as a result of being stimulated by the energy of the sun. This is sometimes manifested as a diffuse darkening like a tan, but chronic and prolonged exposure to the sun eventually causes the pigment cells in specific areas on the face (or any other sun-exposed area such as

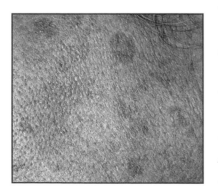

the chest, back, or hands) to break. They then overproduce tan and brown pigment. This creates the discrete oval and round spots called liver spots, age spots, or sunspots, which can be anywhere from one-eighth to three-quarters of an inch in diameter. In addition, the same degree of chronic or repeated sun exposure can cause less discrete, blotchy, uneven brown discolorations, which don't have as sharp a border and can be as large as two or three inches.

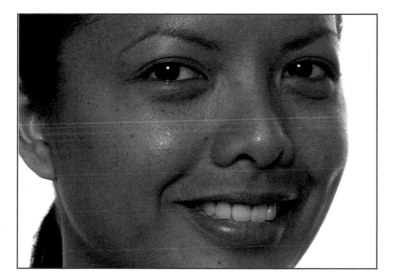

Chloasma (melasma) on upper lip.

Chloasma and melasma are brown, blotchy discolorations of the face, usually seen in women. The cause of both afflictions is female hormones—naturally occurring or occurring as a result of birth control pills. It is common for women to experience these discolorations during pregnancy since female hormones are abundant at that time and can create a photosensitivity—leading to darkening on the forehead or cheeks, around the eyes or the upper lip. Sometimes referred to as "the mask of pregnancy," this brown pigmentation can subside after birth—or after going off the birth control pill—but usually never goes away completely. It is prolonged by breast-feeding. I often recommend skin-bleaching agents and other products such as glycolic acids to aid in the lightening of brown discoloration.

Seborrheic keratoses are the crusty, warty-looking brown growths that commonly appear on skin. They are rough, scaly, raised, greasy-looking growths that vary greatly in size and appearance. They might be smaller than a pencil eraser or larger than a quarter. The color can vary from yellow-tan to brown and black. Seborrheic keratoses are sometimes mistaken for warts, and because they increase in number as we get older, they are sometimes called "senile warts"—but have nothing to do with your state of mind. They are caused by a large number of normal cells (with a normal

Seborrheic keratosis.

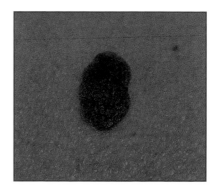

amount of pigment in them) accumulating on the surface of the skin. The extra number of cells alone causes a brown or tan darkening. Seborrheic keratoses occur more frequently from middle age onward, increase in size and number over the years, and are the most common skin growths in adults over the age of forty. They occur primarily on the trunk but are also fairly common on the face, arms, and legs. Heredity commonly contributes to their formation, so look at your parents' skin if you want to look into your future.

Certain lotions and medications, when applied to the skin and then exposed to the sun, can also cause a brown discoloration. These products usually contain oil of bergamot or lemon

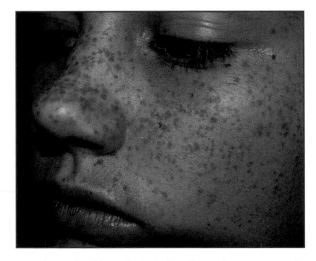

Hereditary freckles, which darken from the sun, on and around the nose.

or lime juice, which all have ingredients that make the skin photosensitive, meaning that the skin overreacts to the energy of the sun and turns brown after being exposed. Some perfumes contain photosensitizers as well.

Freckles contain normal pigment cells that are in the process of making more pigment than usual. The pigment cells are in the bottom layer of the epidermis. These cells have a whole network of dendrites, or tentacles, that extend up into the overlying cells, and they transfer pigment via those dendrites into the cells above. The freckles I am referring to here are the ones you get as a kid based on genetics, and are different from sunspots, age spots, and liver spots, which develop later in life from the degenerative effects of the sun. Freckle pigment cells are easily activated by the sun, leaving you with the visible manifestation of a clustering of normal pigment that is referred to as a freckle. Freckles can be treated by a dermatologist with a series of superficial chemical peels or laser therapy but can return after reexposure to the sun.

Colored or pigmented moles are known medically as *pigmented nevi*. These brownish black colored lesions can appear at any age and grow in various sizes and shapes. The color is caused by the presence of cells (melanocytes) that make and contain melanin, the same pigment responsible for skin color. A mole consists of a discrete aggregation of an increased number of these normal pigment cells. All mole cells are in the epidermis or dermis— the two top layers of your skin. Some moles are flat and look like a freckle; they are referred

NORMAL MOLES VS. DYSPLASTIC NEVI (ABNORMAL MOLES)

	NORMAL MOLES	DYSPLASTIC NEVI
SHAPE	Symmetrical, round, or oval	Often asymmetrical: one half looks obviously unlike the other
BORDER	Regular, sharp, well-defined	Irregular, concave, or hazy; seem to gradually and unevenly fade into the surrounding skin
COLOR	Usually one or two shades of tan, brown, or skin color	Varied (multiple hues) and irregular, with haphazard areas of tan, brown, dark brown or black (sometimes with a pinkish hue)
DIAMETER	Usually less than ¼"; can be covered by a pencil eraser	¼" to ½" or more
LOCATION	Concentrated on sun-exposed skin on the face, trunk, arms, and legs	Most commonly on the back, chest, abdomen, and extremities, but may also occur on normally unexposed areas such as buttocks, groin, and breasts
UNIFORMITY	Resemble one another	Greatly varied; look different from one another
	Normal mole	*Abnormal, irregular, brown mole*

to as *junctional nevi* and are confined to the lower layer of the epidermis. Some moles are raised, some enlarged, and some develop hairs. Moles can change with time, so as you get older they can become elevated and lighter or darker in color; some never change at all. Patients come into my office all the time worried about their raised moles (*intradermal* and *compound nevi*), which can be colored (pigmented) or just skin-colored (not pigmented). The raised mole has a buildup of cells, and it's like a volcano pushing your outer layer of skin (your epidermis) up, although it is solid. Squeezing one of these is like trying to squeeze a brick; whereas a pimple has a semifluid content, a mole never degenerates into fluid.

Moles can darken normally with exposure to the sun, and during puberty and pregnancy, but change in color can also be the first sign that a mole is becoming abnormal and is on its way to becoming cancer (melanoma). If there is a change in a mole's size, shape, or color, or if it bleeds, itches, or becomes painful, immediately contact your dermatologist. Junctional nevi, which look like harmless freckles, can be the most misleading moles since they are the type most likely to turn into skin cancer. Intradermal nevi are dome-shaped and never become skin cancer. Raised moles contain many hair follicles, so they often develop pimples inside, causing a sudden (overnight) and frightening enlargement of the mole. This is nothing to be alarmed by—cancers don't visibly enlarge overnight.

A *compound nevus* is a raised mole made up of a combination of a junctional and an intradermal nevus. And since it is in part made up of a junctional nevus it can also become a melanoma.

The moles most likely to develop into skin cancer are those that are present at birth (*congenital nevi*). The biggest risk comes from congenital moles that measure larger than eight inches in diameter. But moles that develop after birth that are more than 0.6 centimeters in diameter (about the size of a pencil eraser) are also at risk for becoming cancerous.

A *dysplastic mole* may be larger than the average mole, and more irregular in shape. These moles tend to be uneven in color, with dark brown centers and lighter edges. They usually develop sporadically in small numbers during life as a result of intense sun exposure, but in rare cases can occur as a hereditary syndrome. One out of every twenty-five Americans has dysplastic moles. This type of abnormal mole has a 15 to 20 percent lifetime probability of becoming a melanoma and so, in my opinion, should always be removed—even though benign. Because of the potential for all abnormal moles to become melanoma, it's just better not to live with the unnecessary risk.

Post-inflammatory hyperpigmentation (PIH) is a darkening of the skin in response to injury. When the skin is injured it can protect itself in only two ways: darkening or thickening.

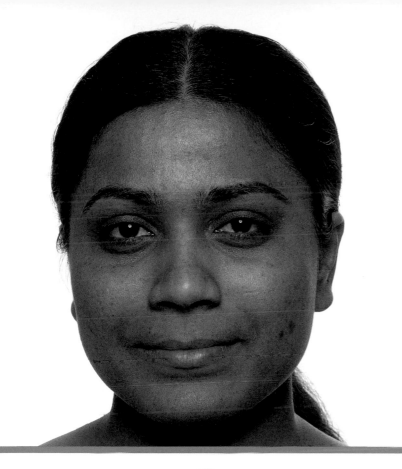

BEFORE: Here we see an example of post-inflammatory hyperpigmentation from acne that has been picked (resulting in larger brown spots than in un-picked pimples), especially on her left cheek (right side of photo).

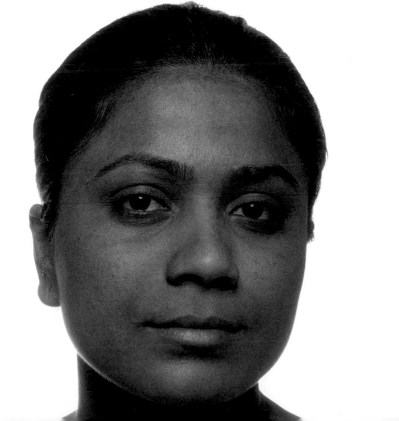

AFTER: Now we observe the complete disappearance of post-inflammatory hyperpigmentation, decreased oiliness, and smaller pores.

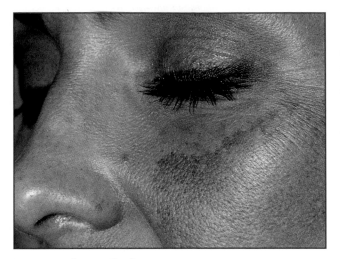
Brown patches on the face.

An example of darkening is a suntan that occurs after a sunburn, which is an injury to the skin. The skin doesn't tan to look beautiful, it tans to protect itself—by preventing additional damaging sunlight, with its harmful UV radiation, from entering the skin. A very common cause of PIH is a burn on the arm from cooking or from touching hot objects. When a burn like this heals, it invariably causes this brown darkening. PIH usually fades over time, and normal skin color returns.

Pityriases alba are round, light patches of the skin. Covered with fine scales, the light patches are the result of mild eczema, and the loss of color is only temporary. The patches, most common in children, can occur anywhere on the body, but are most noticeable on the face and upper arms. See a dermatologist for treatment.

Reds

If you look closely at your face, chances are you will find one or more red spots. Perhaps you've got broken capillaries next to the corner of your nose, or small red dots that just won't go away. Have you ever wondered what those reds are from? Red marks are blood in the skin made visible by enlargement of the tiniest skin blood vessels, which are very superficial, or near the surface of the skin. Their causes are various and include damaging sun radiation, female hormones, pregnancy, physical injury, and alcohol consumption. All of these weaken the vessel walls so the normal pressure of the blood actually stretches them. Then their caliber, or diameter, increases and they carry more blood—and therefore become even larger in size. Our skin, like the rest of our body, has conduits through which the blood travels—arteries, veins, and capillaries.

Most of the redness we see in the skin is an enlargement or engorgement of the little veins (venules) or capillaries, which we call—in both cases—broken capillaries. Broken capillaries have enough blood in them that you can actually see them through the skin. The normal, unaffected capillaries and venules are too small to be seen with the naked eye, but these blood vessels, as a result of their increase in diameter, reach a sufficient size that they are apparent to the naked eye as little red lines, red curves, red bumps, and red blotches. Most people have them on the nose and the cheeks, and although they are usually much less common on the forehead, they can occur anywhere on the face and also on the chest, neck, and legs.

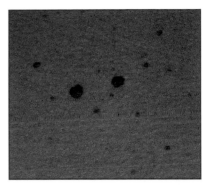

Cherry hemangiomas.

There are basically four types of red lesions, as follows:

Telangiectasias: dilated blood vessels within the skin that appear on the face and are particularly common on the side of the nose. They appear as tiny straight or curved red lines. There are many possible causes including heredity, overexposure to the sun, alcohol consumption, liver damage, pregnancy, normal female hormones, birth control pills, and rosacea. Injuries and even mosquito bites can cause telangiectasias.

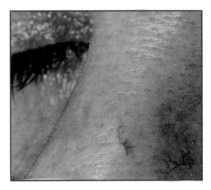

Spider hemangioma across the bridge of the nose.

Cherry hemangiomas: round, tiny (almost always less than an eighth of an inch) bright red flat or dome-shaped sharply bordered spots that occur strictly as a function of getting older in people who inherit a tendency toward them. They increase with age, but they are harmless and only of cosmetic importance. You can literally have hundreds of them.

Spider hemangiomas: small red raised spots with little nonraised red lines emanating from the center like the legs of a spider. When you apply pressure on them with your finger they blanch (lose their red color), and when you release your finger, the center bump visibly refills with blood, then the "legs" do. These are most common on the cheeks of children and often occur as a result of a minor scratch or other injury.

Red blotches or patches: tend to occur on the face (or anywhere on the body in the course of normal healing after an injury). They are made up of a very large aggregation of tiny enlarged blood vessels that are each too small to see with the naked eye but, because of their large number and their being adjacent to each other, together appear as a red blotch or spot.

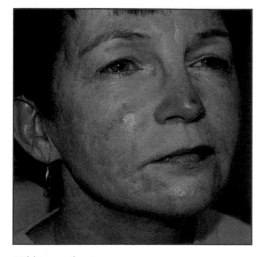

Mild to moderate rosacea.

In addition to these four basic red lesions, several skin conditions are categorized by their annoying and sometimes disfiguring red color.

Rosacea, a chronic disease that affects men and women in their thirties, forties, and fifties, is characterized by redness (blotches or telangiectasias) of the central area of the face due to dilation of small blood vessels. The dilation may be fleeting or long lasting. The condition is sometimes confused with acne because acne-like blemishes are present in addition to the redness. However, an easy way to make the differentiation is to note the absence of blackheads and whiteheads in cases of rosacea. Also, the redness and blemishes are usually confined to the central part (nose and adjoining cheeks) of the face. Rosacea can sometimes cause the oil glands and collagen fibers on the nose to enlarge, resulting in a condition known as rhinophyma. A person affected with rhinophyma develops a big, lumpy, bumpy, very large-pored nose that looks like W. C. Fields's.

The reds that you see *on* the skin are a variation of the reds *in* the skin. Fifty percent of all humans have, from birth, enlarged capillaries on the back of their neck, right under their hair, which are ruby red in color and are called *port-wine stains*. It's remarkably common and normal to be born with this condition. If the port-wine stain is on the face or some other part of the body, it is often referred to as a birthmark, but it is still just a lot of very small enlarged capillaries.

Precancerous actinic keratosis.

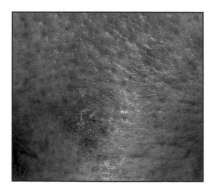

Chronic sun exposure causes a precancerous growth/condition called an *actinic keratosis* or *solar keratosis,* which is a precursor to the middle-grade skin cancer called squamous-cell carcinoma. *Actinic keratosis* most often appears in light-skinned individuals, and is characterized by pink, scaly, rough areas. At the keratosis stage, the area involved is usually less than a half inch in size (or roughly smaller than a dime). This spot develops a persistent rough texture, and is underscored by a pinkish or reddish hue that is based on the degenerative effects of the sun. It is extremely important to have a dermatologist look at any area you suspect to be an actinic keratosis.

More on Blood Vessels

All red defects have to do with blood vessels, but not all red defects are flat, like the ones described above. However, the reds that occur on our facial skin—*the red defects discussed in this book*—are almost all flat: they are either painless, discrete broken capillaries (or telangiectasias), rosacea, a combination of the two, or spider hemangiomas, which can have slightly raised centers.

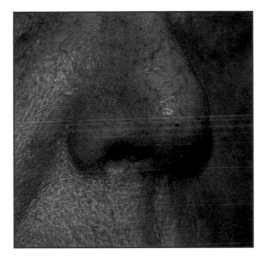

Broken capillaries on the nose. These are also common on cheeks and areas adjacent to the nose.

Reds are difficult to treat with topical ointments. Sulfur is helpful for some redness. Topical cortisone can also be helpful, but you have to use that on a temporary basis or (paradoxically) it can later break capillaries. Reds are not difficult to hide with green-tinted makeup, but it's best to try to *eliminate* red tones whenever possible—something you will learn to do later in this book.

Female hormones, particularly estrogen, have a stimulatory effect on blood vessels, which is important when talking about color ailments because women tend to be more sensitive to these issues than men. Hormone-stimulated growth of the blood vessels results in an increase in their diameter, which causes them to become visible, as explained earlier. Female hormones can cause this dilation of the blood vessels as a result of three different possibilities: First, a woman may just be susceptible (hypersensitive) to hormones—and even a normal hormone level can cause changes in the capillaries. Second, a woman may develop elevated hormone levels; this is natural during pregnancy, as a result of birth control pills, or—less commonly—in the late stages of liver disease. Third, a woman may be receiving the relatively elevated levels of synthetic hormones used for hormone replacement therapy; these are also a factor in blood vessel changes. These conditions span almost the entire lifetime of women, from their teens to their sixties and seventies!

Genetics can also play a role in causing redness of the skin. People of Celtic ancestry have more sensitive skin with less natural protection from the sun; therefore, the damaging effects of the sun are stronger and stand out more in those patients.

Lastly, diet can cause redness in the skin; certain foods have direct dilating effects on the blood vessels. These foods cause the blood vessels to temporarily increase in diameter while the food is in the blood. The most common perpetrators are alcohol and spicy foods—many of us have experienced a temporary reddening or blushing fifteen to thirty minutes after eating these foods. The effect lasts for several hours. Also, certain medications, drugs, and vitamins (the most common of which is any form of niacin, one of the B vitamins) are known to cause dilation of facial blood vessels and therefore to increase their conspicuousness.

African American–related Skin Concerns

Skin color is mostly determined by cells called melanocytes. Within the melanocytes are structures called melanosomes, which produce the pigment melanin. All skin colors have the same number of melanocytes, but black skin's melanocytes have more melanosomes. These melanosomes are also larger than the melanosomes in white skin. Because of their dark skin, African Americans are better protected against skin cancer and premature wrinkling from sun exposure.

However, certain color and texture skin problems are more common among African Americans. For example, *dry skin* is a problem for people of all skin colors, but it may become very distressing to people with black skin. Dry skin in African Americans appears grayish and ashy and is easily noticed because of its obvious difference from the surrounding skin.

Pomades can decrease hair dryness, but can block pores in the scalp, causing the pimples often referred to as pomade acne; this occurs not only in the scalp but also on the face just next to the scalp—the hairline area. (This can happen to anyone, regardless of skin color. Try not to overuse hair products that affect the forehead area.)

Also common among African Americans are the following conditions:

Post-inflammatory hyperpigmentation occurs when an area of the skin darkens after an injury such as a cut or scrape, or in cases of acne. Proper treatment of acne may prevent development of noticeable dark spots, and old dark spots will resolve with time. The best way to prevent post-inflammatory hyperpigmentation is to avoid harsh scrubbing, picking, and abrasive treatments.

Vitiligo is a common condition where pigment cells are destroyed and irregular white spots or patches appear on the skin. The major skin pigment, melanin, is not being produced in certain areas, which causes irregularly shaped white patches to form on the skin. These are most obvious on dark skin but also occur in Caucasians, in whom it is less conspicuous. Vitiligo can occur on any portion of the body. The most common sites are the face, hands, feet, genitalia, and around all body openings. In addition, vitiligo tends to develop in areas that have been injured by cuts, scrapes, or burns. No one knows what causes vitiligo, which affects at least 1 percent of the total population. It is not always easy to cure. The most common method of treatment is medicated creams prescribed by a dermatologist, but if that doesn't work, PUVA therapy—a combination of light treatments and medication—may restore the discoloration. There are also new laser treatments available.

Keloids, or keloid scars, develop when a raised scar from a cut or wound extends and spreads beyond the size of the original wound. These scars vary in shape, size, and location. They are commonly found on the earlobes (from ear piercing), neck, chest, hands, or forearms, and usually occur after an injury or infection. They can also spontaneously occur, especially in the midchest area, but most often follow an injury caused by acne on the chest and back. Depending on the location, keloids can be treated with cortisone injections, pressure, silicone gels, surgery, or laser treatment. Unfortunately, keloids tend to return and even enlarge, especially after treatment with surgery.

TEXTURE

While it is easy to look into a mirror and see color issues on your skin, it isn't possible to feel them. But without ever looking at your skin, you can detect if you have texture issues. When you touch your face, does it feel smooth or rough? Does it feel like the skin of an orange? Can you see flakes of skin on your fingers? Can you feel the undulation of the pores? If there is a lack of "slip factor," or ease, when you run your fingers across your face, you have textural skin problems. Don't feel bad—most of us do.

Textural skin problems consist of the skin being dull, lifeless, or matte in appearance, lacking a luster or glow. In addition, scales or flakes and large pores all contribute to the gestalt of textural problems. I find textural problems to be the most consequential of the three elements of color, texture, and contour.

When thinking about skin texture, imagine a piece of smooth, finished wood next to a

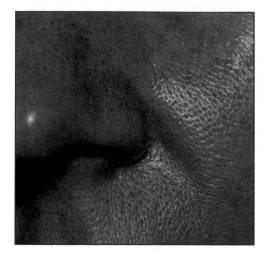
Large pores.

piece of raw, unfinished wood. Unfinished wood is uneven, rough, dull looking, and nonreflective, whereas finished wood is shiny, smooth, and reflective. Painting unfinished wood only makes it look worse; it accentuates the irregularities that characterize unfinished wood. The same holds true for your skin.

Applying makeup on skin with unsatisfactory texture (your uneven, rough, dull exterior) usually *accentuates* and magnifies all of the imperfections and defects. By correcting your texture defects, you can achieve smooth, bright, lively looking skin.

To extend our construction metaphor a little further, your facial skin is also a lot like a shingled roof. As a roof gets older, some of its shingles break or start to turn up at the edges. Those turned-up edges catch unwanted debris, leaves, and twigs. The same thing happens to your cells: You have an infinite number of epidermal cells that lie flat and in register with each other. As you accumulate dead cells, those cells are only being partially shed.

Anything that decelerates the rate of cellular turnover causes you to retain cells, which accumulate in an uneven fashion, causing dull, matte-looking skin. An accelerated cellular turnover causes large flakes, which are cells being shed before they have broken down into smaller, undetectable ones. The skin comes off in strips (like it does when you have a bad sunburn that begins to peel). No doubt about it, dull, matte skin looks tired and less attractive. Not to mention, it is much more difficult to apply makeup to. But the reality is that by the time you get rid of those dead cells and find your new, smooth skin, you won't even need makeup!

Acne

Acne is a disease characterized by a mixture of noninflamed lesions called blackheads (open comedones) and whiteheads (closed comedones), and a variety of inflamed lesions including papules, pustules, cysts, and nodules—what you and I call pimples or zits!

Acne develops in specialized glands called sebaceous follicles. Sebaceous follicles have multiple large oil glands, a very small hair, and a follicular canal, the opening of which is what you recognize as a pore. These follicles are located primarily on the face and, to a lesser extent, on the chest and back. Noninflamed acne begins with an abnormally rapid generation of the cells lining the follicular wall. These cells are normally swept out of the follicle, but in acne the newly generated cells stick together and form a plug, which is invisible from the skin surface. This plug, called a microcomedo, can then enlarge to form a whitehead or a blackhead. In inflammatory acne, bacteria in the follicle release by-products that attract white blood cells (pus) to the follicle. This causes a break in the follicle wall, leading to more inflammation and pimples, which sometimes develop into larger lesions called nodules, or cysts.

The oily material (sebum) secreted by the skin's sebaceous glands is essential in the generation of acne. Without sebum, acne can't occur. Some people believe sunbathing makes acne better—*not true!* In fact, the drying effect is temporary, and UV rays actually stimulate production of oil and thicken the outer layer of skin, which then blocks pores.

Acne is a complex disease, and the degree of control varies. Acne doesn't have to make your life miserable, though, because it is treatable; a skin-care routine such as the one outlined in this book will help minimize the severity of your acne, regardless of its condition.

Enlarged Pores

Another significant texture issue is the presence of large pores. An enlarged pore occurs when the opening of a sebaceous follicular canal is widely dilated. Enlarged pores are most obvious on the nose, lower forehead, chin, and inner aspects of the cheeks, where oil glands are most concentrated. Large pores are caused by swollen, engorged oil glands resulting from the canal being clogged, lending a thick, cobblestoned look to the skin surface. The oil collects in the pores, and dirt from the air gets trapped in the oil, causing little black dots that people mistake for blackheads; the dots are actually just dirt trapped in the oil in the pores. Regular soap just slides over the clogged pores and can't get in to emulsify and pull the oil and dirt out. Large pores really represent an exaggerated enlargement or dilation of the outflow duct from the oil gland. This is an issue that drives many of my patients crazy. Enlarged pores are the antithesis of soft, gentle skin.

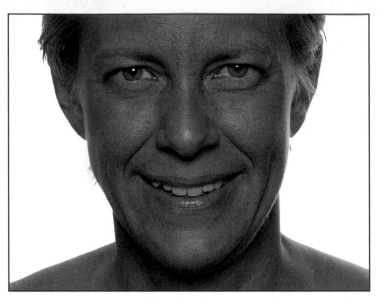

Here's an example of both color (reds) and texture (enlarged pores) problems.

COLOR, TEXTURE, AND CONTOUR COMBINATIONS

Now, you might be wondering if there are any conditions that exist related to color *and* texture *and* contour, and the answer is *yes.* Dark circles under the eyes can be a combination of color, texture, and contour problems. They combine color issues by compounding a darkened brown pigment with enlarged surface red blood vessels called surface capillaries. The red blends with the brown and that, together with the deep blue veins underneath, adds to the dark-circle effect under the eyes. These deep blue veins are called *periocular reticular veins* and are easily treated with laser therapy. Texture and contour issues compound dark circles when you get a puffy appearance under the eye from either swelling or protrusion of the fat pads. This gives the area under your eyes an almost bulged appearance. Those bulges, in turn, cast shadows, contributing to an even darker appearance. Contour issues—fine lines or wrinkles—also contribute to dark circles. The under-eye region is further prone to flaky skin—a textural issue—which only contributes to the darkness.

Finally, you can also get fine lines in the eye area, and when light shines on those lines, the lines cast shadows much like open venetian blinds hanging in front of a window. The program outlined in this book will help you treat dark circles that are caused by fine lines, dry or flaky skin, and brown discoloration.

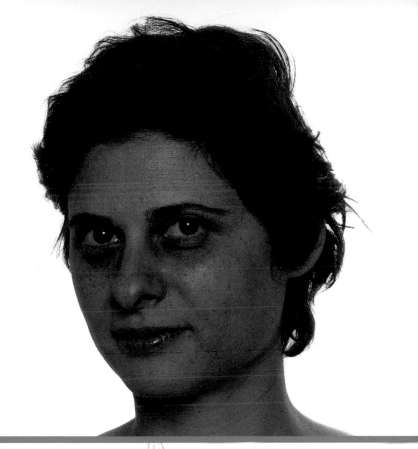

○ BEFORE: **Note the moderate brown discoloration
below the eyes (lower eyelids
and area immediately
adjacent below eyelids).**

○ AFTER: **There's an 80–90
percent reduction in the
brown discoloration of the
lower eyelids and adjacent
area below.**

Now that you know what to look for, take your hand mirror and reexamine your face using only the nonmagnifying side of the mirror. *Use the face diagram provided* or a plain white piece of paper (draw a circle to represent your face) and write down the areas on your face that you think need improvement. The easiest place to start is with color flaws. Color should jump out at you now that you've read all about color issues. Turn your head from side to side and examine your face, ear to ear. Is the color even, or do you see specific areas of different tones? Are there individual areas of drastically different colors? If you see brown spots, are they different shades? Do they have sharp borders, or fuzzy borders? Can you identify red marks? Reds can be more subtle, so look carefully into the mirror, especially when looking for broken capillaries. Sometimes it helps to stretch the skin, especially next to the nose, to find the broken capillaries that run from your cheek onto the wings of the nose. You can stretch the skin right below your eyelids as well since it is more prone to sun damage as a result of the angle. Don't forget to look at your neck and bust area.

Next, look for textural issues by sitting with the light directed at the side of your face—tangential to your skin—while looking into your mirror. This is the easiest (if not the most horrifying) way to look at your skin for texture issues. Search for an absence of luster in your facial skin. Does your skin look dull and lifeless? If you look closer, can you see flakes and scales? Regardless of how the light is coming in, you ought to be able to easily notice any lack of vitality reflecting off your skin. Look for enlarged pores on your nose, cheeks, and the area between your eyebrows. If you can spot black dots, you've got dirt and debris trapped in your pores, and therefore have facial-skin textural issues. See? We all do!

Identify Your Color, Texture, and Contour Flaws

USE THE MAGNIFYING SIDE OF YOUR MIRROR. Again, using either a plain sheet of white paper or the face diagram provided, mark all of the areas you now see that need attention and improvement. Using the diagram, mark all of the areas where you identified color and texture issues. Write down all of the defects you were able to identify by name such as dull areas, broken capillaries, moles, and freckles.

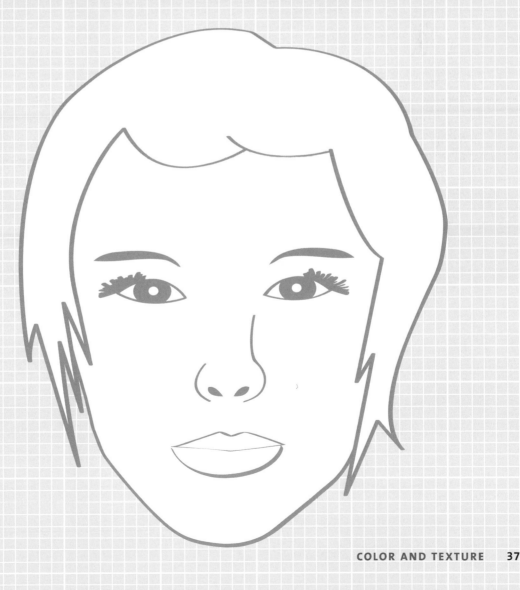

CHAPTER

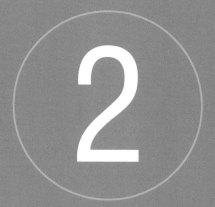

2

*"The expert at anything
was once a beginner."*

HELEN HAYES

Your Skin

LET'S FACE IT, WHEN IT COMES TO OUR SKIN, we know remarkably little about what is going on under the surface. What is our skin made of? And what exactly does it do? These are questions we rarely ask ourselves when looking into a mirror.

There are two main kinds of human skin: nonhairy skin (glabrous skin) and hair-bearing skin. Glabrous skin is found on the palms and soles and is characterized by a thick epidermis. Hair-bearing skin differs from site to site: from the scalp to the arm, for example. It also contains a wide range of other structures depending on the part of the skin examined: Nails are formed from the epidermis on the fingers and toes. Oil glands (sebaceous glands) are found attached to hair follicles. Sweat glands are found in the dermis with ducts passing to the surface through the epidermis. In certain areas such as the axilla (underarm) and groin there are *which weighs 7 pounds (3.2 kg) and has approximately 300 million skin cells. On average each square half inch of skin contains 10 hairs, 15 sebaceous glands, 100 sweat glands, and 3.2 feet (1 m) of tiny blood vessels.*

specialized sweat glands called apocrine glands, which develop after puberty. In addition there are specialized sense organs and nerves, blood vessels and muscles—making the skin one of the most complex organs in the body.

In fact, the brain and skin are deeply connected from the earliest moments of life, and touch is one of the first senses to develop. Even in the womb, a baby feels its way to bring its hand to its mouth. Twenty, thirty, and forty years later, however, it's a different story—we literally lose touch with our skin. When it comes to facial skin, if we see something troubling like a pimple or a discoloration, we give very little thought to how it got there. Let's take a closer look at what exactly makes up our complexions.

WHAT IS SKIN?

Although you may have learned in high school biology about the seven layers of skin, I prefer to talk about the three main layers: the epidermis, the dermis, and the subcutaneous layer. All three play an important part in how the outer surface of the skin appears. It's worth taking a few minutes to learn about and appreciate the dynamic nature of this thing we're in: our skin!

Considering the precious cargo that skin protects, and the endless barrage of factors it protects against, the fact that our skin weighs a mere seven pounds is pretty remarkable. At the surface, skin is a tough outer layer that keeps the body waterproof and sealed off from invaders. Not only does our skin defend against the sun, cold, burns, viruses, and other germs, but it also combats all of the added stress we force upon it with razors, bleaches, hair products, makeup, and abrasive skin-care products—not to mention pollution! The moment its surface is harmed, thereby potentially compromising its barrier function,

FACT: *Humans shed millions of dead skin flakes every day.*

the skin automatically reacts to block infectious germs from getting in and fluids from leaking out. Blood starts clotting and a hyperproduction of skin cells kicks into gear. Flowing toward the center from all sides of the wound, migrating new skin cells eventually meet and multiply until the skin's normal thickness and integrity is restored.

Let's take a look at our first defense against damaging factors: the top layer of skin, the *epidermis*.

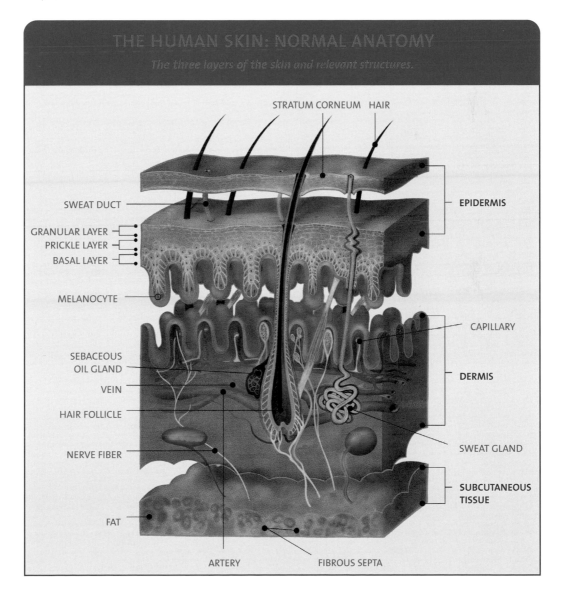

THE HUMAN SKIN: NORMAL ANATOMY

The three layers of the skin and relevant structures.

STRATUM CORNEUM HAIR

EPIDERMIS

SWEAT DUCT

GRANULAR LAYER
PRICKLE LAYER
BASAL LAYER

MELANOCYTE

CAPILLARY

SEBACEOUS
OIL GLAND

DERMIS

VEIN

HAIR FOLLICLE

NERVE FIBER

SWEAT GLAND

SUBCUTANEOUS
TISSUE

FAT

ARTERY FIBROUS SEPTA

The Epidermis

Have you ever thought about how versatile skin is? Mother Nature, genius that she is, equipped our bodies with durability where we need it most and flexibility in the places where it counts. Think about the skin around our eyes: with more than a million tiny movements and blinks a week, the skin here needs to be as flexible and pliable as possible, therefore the skin is only as thick as a single piece of paper. But the soles of our feet, on the other hand, require durability and protection against the brutal beating they take with every step—so the skin there is ten to forty times thicker than the skin on our eyelids. This can be mainly attributed to the first layer of skin—the epidermis—which serves as a protective barrier keeping our inside stuff in and outside stuff out. It keeps infection and pollutants away while holding in fluids, electrolytes, chemicals, clotting factors, and so on. The epidermis is made up of many different layers of cells, like a laminate over a piece of plywood.

> ## HOW THICK IS YOUR SKIN?
>
> *Skin is thickest on the palms and soles (1.2 mm to 4.7 mm) and thinnest on the lips and around the eyes. Facial skin is approximately 0.12 millimeters thick and body skin is about 0.6 millimeters thick.*

The epidermis has four layers within it; from bottom to top they are the basal (or base) layer, the prickle layer, the granular layer, and the horny layer. The horny layer, or *stratum corneum,* is the very outer layer of the skin, and looks (microscopically) like a basket weave; it is thicker in some places—like the soles of our feet—than in others. Although this weave acts as our primary armor against damage, we mostly think of the stratum corneum in negative terms since it is associated with flaky skin or dandruff. Essentially, the horny layer is, in fact, dead skin cells from the epidermis that provide a parting protection before they are sloughed off by our everyday activities. The epidermis is constantly renewing and growing from the bottom upward and the dead skin cells (stratum corneum) are shed, usually invisibly, from the surface.

The rest of our skin's main line of defense from our environment comes from the lower levels of the epidermis—the granular, prickle, and basal layers—which are themselves composed of many layers of multiple cells that make *keratin.* Keratin is the same protein that makes up our hair and nails, which gives you an idea of how tough and protective it can be. The *keratinocyte* cells produce keratin in order to protect the epidermis itself and the layers of skin underneath it, and these little keratin factories make up 95 percent of the total cell count of the epidermis. They are also the origin of most skin cancers, so while they work hard to protect our bodies, they have the potential to be dangerous when something goes wrong.

Keratinocyte cells are created in the basal layer of the epidermis whenever a basal cell divides. Then, for the next fourteen days, the cell travels up through the prickle and granular layers of the skin toward the surface, flattening out as it goes. Finally, the basal cell reaches the surface and then spends another fourteen days flattening out so much that it loses its DNA material and becomes part of the weave of the dead outermost horny layer, ready to be exfoliated (shed). This twenty-eight-day cycle means that the epidermis is constantly renewing itself so that the potential damage perpetually threatening our skin is kept to a minimum.

Making up the other 5 percent of the epidermis are two types of cells: *melanocytes* and *Langerhans cells*. Melanocytes are cells that produce pigment in granules called *melanosomes,* also known as *melanin.* Melanin is a critical molecule manufactured in the melanocytes. Stimulated by sunlight, the melanocytes pump melanin into overlying skin cells by a system of tubes (dendrites) that extend from the melanocyte to the overlying cells. As they migrate up toward the surface, these overlying cells containing melanin help to shield the fragile skin below from the sun.

There is only one melanocyte cell per every ten keratinocytes in the epidermis, and this number holds true regardless of skin color. It is the melanin, the granules within the melanocytes, that determines race or color—according to their size and number. The more melanin, the darker the color of the skin and the greater the protection.

Melanocytes are responsible for the tanning effect we notice when our skin is exposed to the sun's UV rays. In order to protect its nucleus from these damaging rays, the melanocyte reacts by producing larger melanosomes. These melanosomes, under a microscope, look like a shield over the nucleus of the keratinocyte. The darker color we associate with a tan is actually the manifestation of our skin's attempt to protect itself from the mutating and damaging effects of the sun. When the DNA of a melanocyte *is* damaged, it can lead to the development of a deadly skin cancer called melanoma. Bottom line: If your skin is darkened, it's because it has been damaged.

Langerhans cells are part of our diverse immune system, and they reside within the epidermis to alert the system to irritants that cause rashes, like poison ivy. The Langerhans cells monitor the immune reactions and are an important part of our protection against external invasion.

The Dermis

Langerhans cells are not only found in the epidermis, they are also interspersed within the cells of the *dermis,* the skin layer just below the epidermis. The dermis houses miles of blood vessels, bringing nutrients and oxygen to wherever it is needed in the skin.

If the epidermis is like the brick wall around your house—the barrier to the outside world—then the dermis is the mechanical room in your basement. It's where your inner air conditioning is, where your electricity comes from, and where your blood vessels, oil glands, sweat glands, and nerves are. The dermis is thicker than the epidermis: it can reach three millimeters in depth on areas like the back. Compared to the epidermis, the dermis comprises a large percentage of the skin because it provides the main ingredient for holding skin together. It is also the site for most of the specialized functional parts of the skin that make it such a dynamic organ.

The main structural component of the dermis is *collagen.* You've probably heard about collagen on television advertisements for antiwrinkle creams, but you might not know that this versatile protein is *everywhere* in our bodies. It makes up three-quarters of the dry weight of our skin, and it is also found in our tendons, ligaments, and the lining that covers our bones. Its durability is what makes collagen so important—and when this durability gives out from constant damage, we all want our collagen restored in order to reverse the effects of wrinkling and sagging skin.

> ALMOST 2 MILLION YEARS AGO,
> early humans developed a roving way of life and needed a different skin to go with it. It took 1 million years, but humans eventually lost their thick coat of fur, and their sweat glands multiplied, creating an ingenious system that allows them to dissipate heat faster than any other mammal.

Collagen is produced by cells in the dermis called *fibroblasts.* The fibroblasts make collagen in long chains. Then the collagen is dispersed to heal skin wounds; it is a building block for new skin production because of its strength—much of scar tissue is, in fact, collagen. Because collagen is produced in the dermis, it is an important factor in scarring: scar tissue is only created when the depth of an injury extends through the full thickness of the epidermis and into the dermis. If the injury does not affect the dermis, scarring does not occur, because the epidermis is able to completely repair and regenerate itself. But if a wound does extend into the dermis, new collagen is made and sent to the scene, and scarring inevitably occurs.

Collagen's main partner in helping to maintain the skin is a protein called *elastin*. Elastin's purpose is to provide—no big surprise here—elasticity to the skin. How often do *you* sleep on your side with your face scrunched into the pillow? And how often do you see people walking around with their face permanently scrunched? Never, I hope, and that is because of elastin. Elastin gives the skin its invaluable distensibility and accompanying elasticity, and helps maintain skin's shape even after it's been stretched or pulled. The fine filaments of protein that make up elastin help the skin to bounce back and snap into place, but as many of us know all too well, elastin's elasticity wears out over time. Prolonged sun exposure and harsh treatment of the skin break down the coiled filaments of elastin so that, like an overused rubber band, they break and can no longer function normally. This leads to loose and sagging skin.

The dermis is not just filled with proteins. Besides collagen and elastin, the dermis contains many different glands that secrete vital fluids. The dermal *apocrine glands,* located especially in the armpits and nipples, produce and secrete fluids called pheromones. Pheromones are scentless until they interact with bacteria at the skin's surface; this interaction creates a scent that is unique to every individual.

Along with the apocrine glands in the dermis are *sweat glands*. These glands provide a critical, life-sustaining service for the body: they cool us down. While blood vessels contract and expand within the dermis to help regulate body temperature, the millions of coiled sweat glands discharge sweat and salts to the skin surface, where evaporation can begin to cool the body in seconds. Both of these mechanisms permit the skin to disperse heat when necessary, keeping the fragile human engine from overheating.

Without sweat, our body temperatures would rise dangerously high, and we would die. Even the tiny ridges of a fingertip harbor sweat glands. The trigger for how much sweat is released by a single sweat gland is a nerve fiber called a *cholinergic fiber,* and it responds to heat and to emotional stress to affect when and how much we sweat to cool ourselves down.

Sebaceous glands also find their home in the dermal layer of skin. Sebaceous glands are responsible for secreting oils to lubricate hair and the skin itself. Have you ever noticed that the skin on your forearms rarely gets dry, but the skin on your legs can become irritated and flaky without moisturizer after shaving? That's because hair is what disperses the oil from the sebaceous gland. Take away the hair, and the sebaceous gland is less effective. Humans are covered with hair, about five million follicles on average, but thankfully it's more fluff than fur.

The dermis goes well beyond functioning as an inner thermostat. It is also very rich in blood vessels, lymph channels, and nerves—integrating the skin into the vast immune, circulatory, metobolic, and nervous systems of our bodies.

The Subcutaneous Layer

The bottom, or third, layer of skin is called the *subcutis,* or *subcutaneous layer.* The word *cutis* simply means "skin." The subcutis, then, is technically the layer *underneath* the skin, but it is actually considered a part of skin because it is not part of the muscular system below. The subcutaneous layer acts as an energy reserve and an important insulating layer, and provides cushioning and protection. It is mostly made up of fat cells called *lipocytes* that are held together by collagen bands. This layer gives us our own particular shapes, because unlike the epidermis and the dermis, the subcutaneous layer has no limit to how thick it can be. The lipocytes here get most of their press time under another name: cellulite.

Cellulite is the puckered appearance of the skin over normal deeper fat deposits. The bands of collagen that divide the fat cells cause cellulite as they pull from the base of the subcutis to the surface of the skin. It's a lot like the ties used in finishing a quilt: the fibrous bands of collagen act like thread that pulls the puffy insides of the quilt (or in this case, our thighs!) down in the middle creating the unsightly puckered appearance of cellulite.

> ### WHERE ARE THE OIL GLANDS?
>
> *There are 400 to 900 oil glands per square centimeter on the face, but only 100 per square centimeter on the rest of the body! The only areas of skin that do not have any oil glands are the palms of the hands and the soles of the feet.*

With a little knowledge of what's normally going on under the surface of our skin, we can better assess when things go wrong, and deal appropriately with the visible effects. It cannot be stressed enough, however, that no one knows more about skin than a dermatologist—so when in doubt, get it checked out.

FACT: *The human body creates a new layer of skin every 28 days.*

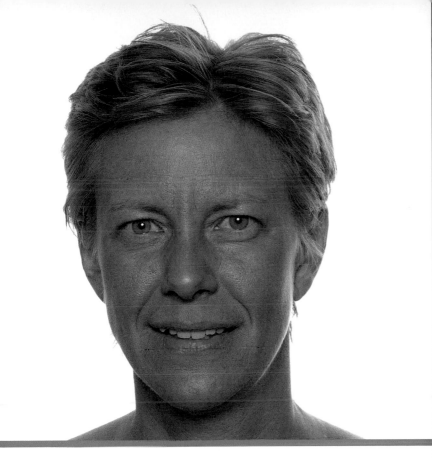

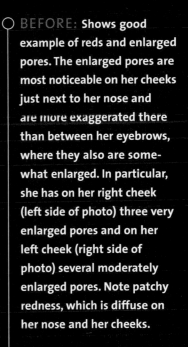

BEFORE: Shows good example of reds and enlarged pores. The enlarged pores are most noticeable on her cheeks just next to her nose and are more exaggerated there than between her eyebrows, where they also are somewhat enlarged. In particular, she has on her right cheek (left side of photo) three very enlarged pores and on her left cheek (right side of photo) several moderately enlarged pores. Note patchy redness, which is diffuse on her nose and her cheeks.

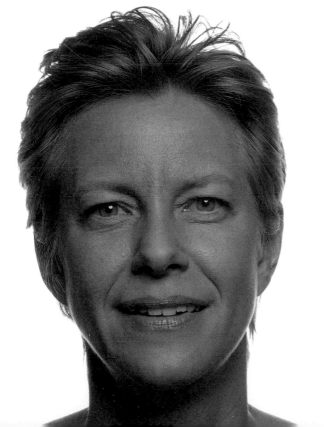

AFTER: Shows marked reduction in redness and improved texture. Her skin just looks smoother, with a significant reduction in pore size next to the nose (on both sides) and a somewhat less dramatic improvement in pore size between the eyebrows. Also, her skin is less oily and the oil and water are in better balance.

CHAPTER

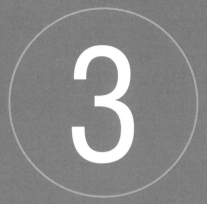

3

*"How old would you be if you
didn't know how old you was?"*

LEROY "SATCHEL" PAIGE

Your Skin Type

○

THE IMPORTANCE OF SKIN TYPES

PATIENTS OFTEN COME INTO MY OFFICE complaining their skin is too oily and too dry. And then they say, "But that's impossible. It can't be oily and dry at the same time," or they complain of their skin being too sensitive. Rarely do they have it right. Patients sometimes think that oil and water are opposites of each other—which they are not. Patients who complain of sensitive skin usually just can't find the correct products for their skin because they don't know or understand their skin type. Most people who think they have sensitive skin really don't. But using the wrong products for your skin type will either fail to fix your problem, or worse, aggravate it—erroneously leading you to believe you have sensitive skin.

In order to lay out an effective skin-care regimen, it is paramount to first determine your specific skin type. There are two distinct categories of skin type: the cosmetic, or facial-skin type, and the Fitzpatrick skin type. Everyone has a cosmetic type *and* a Fitzpatrick type— and the two types tell you remarkably different things about your skin and how you should be treating it. For the purposes of choosing correct and effective skin-care products, it's the cosmetic, or facial-skin type, that is critical.

COSMETIC, OR FACIAL-SKIN TYPES

Cosmetic, or facial-skin types are determined by the relative balance between oil and water in and on your skin. There are six different types of skin that fall under the cosmetic-type category: normal, oily/acne-prone, dry, combination, mature, and sensitive. More detailed information about each type will follow, but first here's a brief description of each type and its relation to the oil-and-water-balance table.

Normal skin occurs when the net result of the oil and water in and on your skin is normal and in balance. Oily/acne-prone skin occurs when the oil glands overproduce, creating more oil than normal. Dry skin happens when water glands are not producing enough water. Combination skin is both dry and oily in different places at the same time. Mature skin is older skin with underproductive oil glands, accompanied by less water content and/or retention, so the skin is extra dry. Sensitive skin can be normal in terms of oil and water balance, but is easily irritated by many common skin-care products.

There are many ways to determine your facial-skin type. Quizzes and questionnaires abound on the Internet about the state of your skin during different times of the day, month, and year; about the way stress affects your skin; about the reaction your skin has to certain products and to certain activities; and about any number of other specific environmental factors. But many of the quizzes available on the Internet are inaccurate, even blending questions about Fitzpatrick skin types with questions about cosmetic/facial-skin types. There is no logic behind these mixed questions since these skin types are not the same.

The easiest way to determine—at least roughly—your skin type is to conduct a very simple test in the privacy of your own home. The only equipment you need is some water and a tissue or brown paper bag. Perform the test at least an hour after washing your face—but before putting any products on your skin. Use the tissue or bag and press your entire face

OIL-AND-WATER-BALANCE CHART

WATER CONTENT OF SKIN	INCREASED OIL	DECREASED OIL	NORMAL OIL
NORMAL	Oily/Acne prone	Doesn't exist	Normal
DECREASED	Combination	Mature	Dry
INCREASED	Doesn't exist	Doesn't exist	Doesn't exist

with it. Make sure to blot your forehead, chin, cheeks, and nose. If skin particles appear on the tissue or bag, or you can see flakes or scales on your cheeks, you have *dry* skin. If you have acne or some areas (mainly the forehead and nose) leave an oily residue on the tissue or bag, but other areas (like the cheeks) do not, you have *combination* skin. If you have acne or all areas leave an oily residue, you have *oily* skin. If you are older and your entire face has scales, flakes, or appears to thirst for water, you have *mature* skin. And if there is no oily residue or skin flakes, and you are not prone to acne, you have *normal* skin.

Knowing your skin type will allow you to troubleshoot any problems that pop up, such as a breakout or flaky skin. It will also help you choose skin-care products more effectively. The three real issues to consider when determining your skin type are oil, water, and sensitivity. Oil is a material made by your oil glands; in its proper quantity, it is barely detectable. Water is made by your sweat glands; as long as you have enough of it, you don't notice anything out of the ordinary, and your skin feels normal. Sensitivity refers to irritation from many common topical preparations—products that are easily tolerated by most people but that irritate sensitive skin. Irritation can occur as a burning or stinging sensation or as redness on the skin.

Dry skin and oily skin are at the two opposite ends of the skin-type spectrum; if you read carefully about both types, you will be able to pinpoint which of the six categories your skin falls into and go from there when choosing products. If you hold up your hand mirror and examine your facial skin closely, can you tell your skin type simply by sight? Use your fingers and feel your skin. Is it greasy feeling? Dry and flaky? How has your skin historically responded to different products? All of these questions factor in to understanding your skin type, and everything we do together from this point forward is predicated on determining your skin type. Once you know that, you will be able to find the right products to fix the color and texture issues that brought us together in the first place. And *that* is a promise.

Normal Skin

Your skin is considered normal if your face is not oily, dry, or sensitive. Normal skin has small pores and is smooth to the touch. Most people have normal skin, which is not to say that most people never have troubling breakouts or times when their skin could use a little extra moisture. Having normal skin simply means that the water and oil in and on your skin are in balance, so your skin does not react negatively to products or external factors, and does not break out excessively. If your skin does not feel flaky or look dry, if you don't have puddles of oil coming from your pores, or an unusual sheen at 11:00 A.M., and if oil isn't breaking through your makeup, then you probably have normal skin. In terms of a skin-care program, normal skin reacts best to gentle, non-soap cleansing, and a light, oil-free moisturizer.

Oily/Acne-prone Skin

Now that you know what *doesn't* constitute an oil imbalance, here are the things that do. If you *do* break through with oiliness two hours after washing, or you literally see oil filling or exuding from your pores, especially in the T-zone (the area across your forehead, nose, and chin), you have excess oil. If your pores always seem enlarged, they have these little black specks in them that you can't get out, or you have frequent breakouts of acne and a tendency to have lots of blackheads (closed comedones) or whiteheads (open comedones), then you have oily skin.

Oily or acne-prone skin tends to be considered a curse—but relax, I assure you it is not. Overproductive oil glands and normal water content give your skin an excessive sheen and an oily feel, often leading to acne. Pores are generally large and open, and skin is coarse and subject to blackheads. However, it can be argued that having oily skin is actually a good thing, because it means that as you grow older, as your skin eventually loses its natural water retention, the oil you produce will help retain moisture. The great advantage, then, is that oily skin ages at a slower rate than other skin types. It's like trading pimples for wrinkles.

Oily skin is caused by many factors. Heredity, hormone levels, pregnancy, birth control pills, cosmetics, and the weather all weigh in. It is true that the hormonal shifts of adoles-

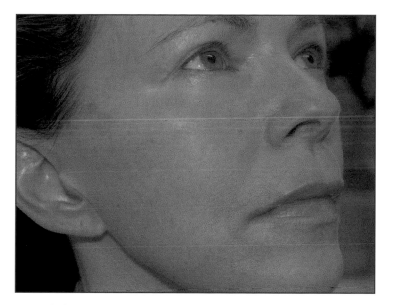

Normal skin.

cence sometimes stimulate sebaceous glands into producing more oil, but oily or acne-prone skin is not simply a teenage problem; the shiny skin that used to be associated uniquely with adolescence today follows women and men into their twenties, thirties, and even beyond. During pregnancy and menopause, for example, hormonal imbalances increase the activity of sebaceous glands and the resulting acne can almost drive peri-menopausal women to drink.

When choosing products for oily skin, detergent-based soaps are not encouraged. While these products may claim to specifically target excess oil, the overdrying effect is incredibly harsh and can sometimes trigger oil glands to produce even more oil as an attempt to protect skin from potential damage. This reaction is called *reactive seborrhea,* and occurs when oil glands work overtime to compensate for the loss of natural oils. Also to be avoided are products that leave the skin feeling taut. This drying causes the upper layers of skin to shrink, restricting oil flow through the pores, which leads to blockages and breakouts.

When deciding on a moisturizer (or any skin-care product), look for one that is labeled *water based, oil free,* or *noncomedogenic*. Otherwise, don't even think of using it, unless, of course, it says *for oily skin*. Remember to use a lotion and not a cream. Lotions are lighter and tend to contain less oil, so they won't clog pores and lead to an acne outbreak. Oil-free sunscreens are readily available, so you can protect yourself from sun damage without adding extra shine or aggravating or causing acne.

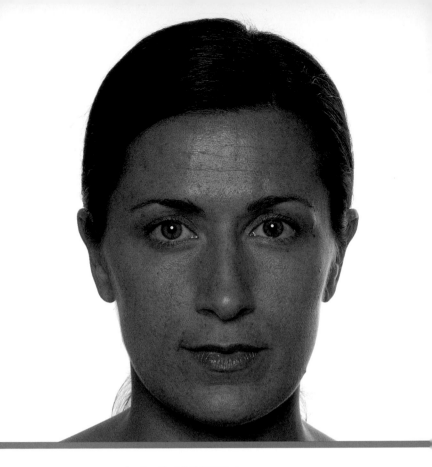

BEFORE: Very oily skin, active pimples on the chin and forehead, and multiple spots of increased pigmentation on the forehead from previous acne lesions. In addition, there are large pores on the cheek areas next to the nose as well as the area between the eyebrows and above the nose. Underground pimples are evident on her left chin. Also, on her forehead, above her right eyebrow, depressions are apparent where pimples have been scratched.

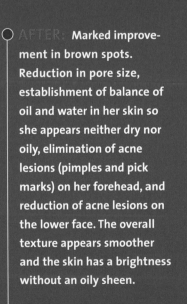

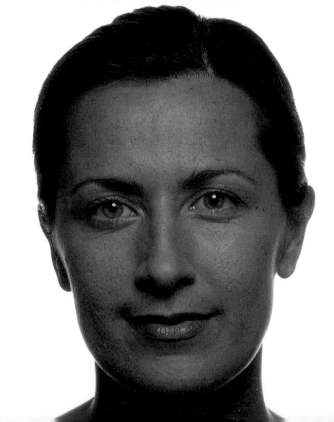

AFTER: Marked improvement in brown spots. Reduction in pore size, establishment of balance of oil and water in her skin so she appears neither dry nor oily, elimination of acne lesions (pimples and pick marks) on her forehead, and reduction of acne lesions on the lower face. The overall texture appears smoother and the skin has a brightness without an oily sheen.

Dry Skin

Dull-looking, flaky, scaly skin, especially on your cheeks, is generally a telltale sign of dry skin. This is because your oil glands (which are fewer in number on your cheeks than on your T-zone) make a normal amount of oil, but your water glands do not produce enough water. Dry skin feels tight after cleansing, and is characterized by small pores or a pinched look. Chapping and cracking are signs that you have extremely dry skin. However, it's rare to develop dry skin in the T-zone area, since you have a higher concentration of oil glands in that area that coat the skin and keep your natural moisture from easily evaporating. If you see flaking in your T-zone, it's probably related to an oil-gland problem (causing inflamed skin and flakiness) rather than to dry skin—unless you are over forty-nine, in which case it might be a sign of mature skin.

Flakiness that you see as a result of dry skin causes a dull, matte appearance. Individual dry flakes of skin stick up, causing them to contract and pull away from the underlying normal skin. This is different from piles of flakes, which is caused by more compact cells that form mini-mounds all over your face, creating other textural issues. With dry skin, the flakes are just one flake thick and uniform. Both *flaking* and *dry-skin flakiness* have the net effect of causing a dull or matte appearance, but only flakes caused from dry skin are relevant in determining your skin type.

> NOT EVERY FLAKE OF SKIN *is an indication of dry skin. Flaking or scaling skin is a final common pathway, the result of many conditions including seborrhea, dandruff, eczema, and sunburns.*

Flakes, in general, are associated with dry skin; however, it is important to note that flakiness is actually a final common pathway from many different medical conditions—particularly from inflammation of the skin. Many people with normal skin develop dry skin during the winter months, when their skin is exposed to the elements. Dryness is exacerbated by wind and extremely low temperatures and low humidity—components of cold air. Cold, dry air causes moisture on the skin to evaporate, and wind accelerates the process, contributing to overdrying of skin. Exposure to the sun also has a drying effect, as does using certain cosmetics, harsh soaps, hot water, or bathing excessively. Dry skin can also be a sign of other health conditions, so if your skin seems abnormally dry, be sure to check with your dermatologist for dermatitis, eczema, psoriasis, or seborrhea. An underactive thyroid can also cause dry skin, as can certain drugs like antihistamines, diuretics, and antispasmodics.

Combination Skin

Combination skin is both oily and dry simultaneously. It's a two-for-one special—lucky you! Overproductive oil glands in the T-zone and underproductive water glands in the cheeks cause this skin type. Caring for combination skin is simply about getting all the zones of your face back in balance.

To restore your skin's natural balance, you need to remove the excess oil *without* removing the water. It's a bit of a slippery slope since in your zeal to remove the excess oil, it can be easy to further overdry your cheeks. If in the process of removing the excess oil from the T-zone you in fact remove necessary water from the cheek area, you will then need to restore that moisture again with an oil-free or water-based moisturizer. But keep in mind that you don't necessarily need to return moisture to the T-zone; in fact, using moisturizer only where you need it is the best route for people with combination skin.

The only thing more difficult than addressing combination skin is addressing combination skin in people who also have sensitive skin. In these rare cases, three different skin types simultaneously converge. But because this book can't be all things to all people, I encourage those of you who think you have this rare skin combination to seek professional help in caring for your skin.

Mature Skin

Mature skin is the only skin type that is truly correlated with age. It occurs as the result of the natural aging process, which causes underactivity of both oil and water glands. As a result, skin is diffusely dry, rough, lacking sheen, and matte. It has an almost leathery quality. Mature skin acts very much like dry skin, and should be treated as such, with extra attention paid to mild but effective exfoliation to increase cell turnover and to refresh the skin's appearance. (In my office we expedite this process with stronger glycolic acid treatments.)

Normally, oil helps protect, lubricate, soften, and add sheen to your skin—and helps skin retain water for normal moisture. But in mature skin, the naturally occurring loss of oil glands (and corresponding loss of oil) and the underactive water glands result in dull skin. Thankfully, though, you can have satisfactory control over the dryness of your skin by replacing the decreased amounts of oil and water with appropriate moisturizers and oil-based or oil-containing products.

Mature skin is typically skin that is beginning to show many signs of aging: fine and medium lines and wrinkles, broken blood vessels and capillaries, roughness, thinning of all three layers of the skin, discoloration, and deep wrinkling. It can sometimes look translucent, almost becoming a window into the deeper layers of the skin, because of the thinning of all your skin layers. That's why you can see broken capillaries and veins more easily in older skin. Mature skin is very fragile because the upper epidermal layer, which is the barrier—or protective—layer of skin, has diminished; and both the middle dermal layer, which is the structural layer, and the lower fat layer are thinning.

The best way to prevent the signs of aging skin is to minimize exposure to the extrinsic, or external, causes of visible skin aging. The sun is the main source of extrinsic aging—and it is never, ever, too late for the protective benefits of sunscreen.

Mature skin benefits greatly from the application of products with "actives" such as alpha- or beta hydroxy acids, which can make mature skin look decades younger and healthier. These products will be discussed at length later on, but it is important to note that many moisturizers contain these ingredients, which, as long as they have excellent moisturizing additives, are recommended for people with mature skin. In fact, to accommodate the increasing number of people with mature skin, three of the six moisturizers in my skin-care line are formulated exclusively for mature skin.

Sensitive Skin

Sensitive skin, regardless of its oil or water content, is easily irritated by many common skin-care products and cosmetics and by the environment. It is typically itchy and variably inflamed (pink, red, scaly, or crusty). Certain foods, and just about anything that comes into contact with the skin, can cause flare-ups; therefore, the fewer products you use—with the fewest ingredients—the better. That way you are minimizing the chances of a negative reaction. Any product you do use should be fragrance free, dye free, and hypoallergenic. Fragrance is the leading cause of contact allergy from topically applied products, but there are many, many products available that are fragrance free. Other topical irritants to be avoided are preservatives, alpha hydroxy acids, tretinoin, salicylic acid, vitamin E, lanolin, fabric softeners, fragranced clothing detergents, and essential oils. Avoid using toners and astringents unless they are alcohol free. Sensitive skin is, unsurprisingly, hypersensitive to the ultraviolet rays of the sun, so an effective sunblock

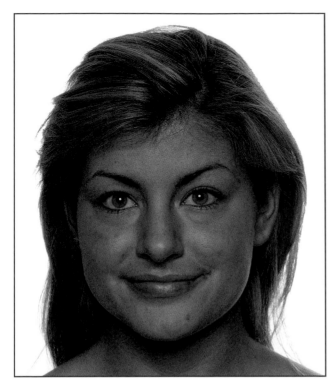

Diffuse blotchy redness is very common in easily irritated sensitive skin.

(SPF 30) is encouraged in a cream or lotion vehicle; gels and alcohol-based products are too irritating.

In determining and describing the skin you are in, facial-skin type is only one piece of the puzzle. The other is not determined by how oily or dry your skin is, but by how easily your skin burns and is thereby damaged—leading to premature wrinkling, age spots, and skin cancer. This second categorization is the Fitzpatrick skin type.

FITZPATRICK SKIN TYPES

The six types of skin defined as Fitzpatrick skin types were first characterized by Thomas Fitzpatrick, M.D., professor emeritus of dermatology at Harvard University. The same vulnerability that predisposes you to sunburn also predisposes you to skin cancer and premature wrinkling of the skin. The fairer your skin, the greater your risk. Determining your Fitzpatrick type is all about assessing skin-cancer risk factors as well as predicting vulnerability to and thereby prevention of premature and unnecessary photoaging, which manifests as many forms of degenerative sun damage including premature wrinkling, sun/age spots, broken capillaries, cobblestoning, dullness, enlarged pores, and decreased elasticity.

Type I skin never tans—it always burns—and it freckles easily. Type I skin is Caucasian (as are types II, III, and IV), and people with this type of skin have red or blond hair and blue or green eyes. *Type II* skin is very similar to type I, in that it is fair and white and freckles

FITZPATRICK SKIN TYPES

SKIN TYPE	NATURAL SKIN COLOR	RESPONSE TO SUN EXPOSURE
I	Caucasian	Always burns, never tans
II	Caucasian	Usually burns, tans minimally
III	Caucasian	Burns minimally, tans gradually, uniformly
IV	Caucasian	Burns minimally, always tans well
V	Light brown (Asian and Hispanic)	Rarely burns, tans darkly
VI	Dark brown (African American)	Never burns, tans darkly

easily, but it is slightly less sensitive to the sun and is borne by people with a broader range of eye colors, including hazel and brown. While this skin type burns easily, it can, with some effort, tan lightly. *Type III* skin usually tans lightly instead of forming discrete freckles, and only burns occasionally. People with type III skin have white skin and blond or brown hair. *Type IV* skin almost always tans darkly and rarely burns. This skin is usually Caucasian, naturally darker or light brown, and people with this skin type tend to have brown or black hair. *Type V* skin (often Hispanic or Asian) is naturally light brown and always tans. People with type V skin have brown or black hair and eyes. *Type VI* skin is brown or black, and tans are difficult to see. People with type VI skin (African Americans) also have black hair and brown eyes. Type VI skin carries the lowest risks for skin cancer, due to the inherent protection from the sun's damaging UV rays afforded by dark, deeply pigmented skin.

The Fitzpatrick skin types can be broadly regarded as generally grouping skin types according to ethnic origins. Types I and II tend to belong to people from Celtic (Scotch-Irish),

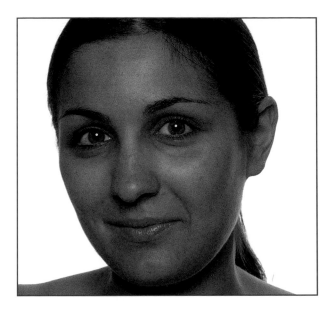

TOP: *TYPE V SKIN: I consider this a "pretty" example of type V skin. No specific lesions or defects demonstrable here.*

BOTTOM: *TYPE VI SKIN: A good example of type VI skin. In addition, her facial skin type is normal.*

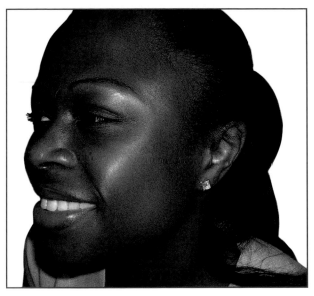

Scandinavian, or Northern European backgrounds; types III or IV to people from Mediterranean backgrounds—Italians, Spaniards, and Greeks. East Asians and Hispanics are generally type V, and sub-Saharan Africans and African Americans, type VI. But ethnicities' evolution and variation mean that regardless of your background, determining your own specific skin type—using the above type categories as well as your own history in responding to sun exposure—is crucial to evaluating your needs and risks. In short, Fitzpatrick skin types represent a scale of the skin's photosensitivity, which will help in deciding which sunscreens to use, and how best to protect yourself from all types of sun damage—from wrinkles to precancers to actual skin cancer.

Once you determine your two skin types—facial and Fitzpatrick—it will be easy to choose a line of skin-care products that will cleanse, rejuvenate, moisturize, protect, and benefit your skin in the best way possible.

What's Your Skin Type?

CIRCLE ALL THAT APPLY.

1. In the past three months, I have had pimples, blackheads, whiteheads, or undersurface bumps on my face, and/or oily skin.

2. The skin on my cheeks, but not around my nose or between my eyebrows, is dry, flaky, or tight.

3. I'm "of a certain age"—the skin of my entire face, including my T-zone (forehead, nose, and chin) is dry, flaky, scaling, or thirsting for moisture and very difficult to keep moisturized.

4. Many different common skin-care products easily irritate my facial skin causing redness, a burning sensation, stinging, pain, and/or swelling.

5. My facial skin is neither prone to pimples, blackheads, whiteheads, or undersurface bumps nor dry or easily irritated by different skin-care products.

If the following numbers are circled, then your skin type is as indicated:

1: acne prone / oily	**1 & 4:** acne prone / oily and sensitive
2: dry	**2 & 3:** mature
3: mature	**2 & 4:** dry and sensitive
4: sensitive	**3 & 4:** mature and sensitive
5: normal	**1, 2, & 4:** combination and sensitive
1 & 2: combination	**2, 3, & 4:** mature and sensitive

Your skin should fall into one of the above categories, which represent the only logical combinations for determining skin type.

CHAPTER

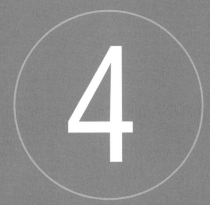

4

*"An ounce of prevention
is worth a pound of cure."*

PROVERB

How Your Skin Got Where It Is

THE SECOND YOU STEP ON A SCALE and the number is bigger than you expected, you know that something has to change. But you usually don't really need a scale to tell you that. It's obvious: Your clothes are too tight. You easily become winded. All the telltale signs are there that something is wrong. Should you go on a high-protein, low-carbohydrate diet? Should you go on The Zone? Maybe you want to give the South Beach Diet or Atkins a try? Perhaps it's time to use that home gym you bought last year—the one that serves as a place to hang winter coats. How does anyone know for sure what program will work for them? They don't. What they do know, without a doubt, is that they are overweight. Something is wrong and it needs to be fixed.

That's how I think most people feel when looking at their facial reflection. They know something is wrong, but are completely at a loss as to the proper course of action for attaining a brighter, healthier reflection.

If we never exposed our skin to the sun's damaging effects of photoaging, our aging faces would only be caused by two things: loss of elastic tissue, which is in the dermis layer of the skin, and loss of fat. We would have no color issues, and barring any genetic failure, pretty good texture. But even someone whose skin has never been abused by the sun still ages and therefore loses elasticity in the skin. It is an inevitable reality for all of us.

Loss of elasticity in the skin happens from sun exposure and plain chronologic aging. When elastic fiber is lost, the skin sags in response to the immutable forces of gravity. Interestingly, the loss of elastic fibers has very little effect on texture or color; it mostly affects contour. While it is possible to restore collagen in the skin by either injecting it or by using glycolic acids or tretinoin (Retin A), there is no way to restore elastic tissue. Once it's gone, it's gone.

Three things cause the loss of elastic tissue. First, the natural aging process. Second, ultraviolet radiation from the sun—which is the best way to prematurely lose your elastic tissue and thereby prematurely wrinkle your face. Smoking certainly aggravates the situation and is the second-best way to spoil your skin. Third, elastic failure. Much like on an old pair of underwear, when the skin has been repeatedly stretched, the elastic just gives out and doesn't have the same tension. Elastic fibers have a limited number of stretches before their elasticity breaks and they stop working.

That's why I would caution you against creams claiming to reduce or eliminate wrinkles for four to six hours; what these creams are really doing is causing a temporary swelling and thereby a stretching of the elastic fibers—and once that swelling goes down, your wrinkles come back. If you reapply the cream, all you are really doing is making a bad situation worse by creating undue repeated stretching of already damaged elastic fibers and further shortening their useful life by using up their limited number of lifetime stretches. If you want permanent bags and sagging, keep using those so-called magic creams. Like in dieting, where everyone is looking for that instant-cure magic pill, there is no magic cream, ointment, lotion, or potion when it comes to skin care—and especially when it comes to lines and wrinkles.

TIME IS A GREAT HEALER BUT A LOUSY BEAUTICIAN

Aging of the skin is an inevitable and irreversible result of passing time, aggravated by damage from the sun. Unless you're already dead (and therefore probably not reading this book) you are aging. After age twenty-five, collagen fibers in the dermis begin to break down, subcutaneous fat begins to gradually disappear, and skin becomes drier and holds less water. Cumulative years of the downward pull of gravity and of our elastic fibers breaking or withering away lead to sagging skin and wrinkles.

There are essentially two kinds of aging: intrinsic and extrinsic. Intrinsic aging of the skin happens as a result of time and genetics. Time is nature's way of keeping everything from happening at once. Genetics is nature's way of saying you can run, but you can't hide. Think of your facial skin like a circus tent with poles holding up the periphery. The big top is in the center, and it has a much taller pole, which gives the height in the center of the tent. Loss of collagen, to some extent, makes the big top fall in. But loss of fat will make that big top fall all the way down to the ground. Until the apples from Newton's tree rise magically from the ground back up to the branches, and until people start walking on their hands with their feet up in the air, we will always have the issue of gravity-driven falling skin. Loss of collagen causes lines and wrinkles. Loss of fat causes furrows and troughs. By then, the big top is on the ground—all caved in.

Extrinsic aging of the skin is caused by the sun, smoking, and all other external forces your skin is exposed to every day, causing many of your face's color, texture, and contour problems. There are three inexorable factors that will impact your facial skin whether you want them to or not: time, genetics, and the sun. Together, they deviously account for the intrinsic and extrinsic aging of your skin that causes you to have a bad mirror day. But don't worry: the information in this book will help you have and keep the skin you've always wanted—forever!

Genetics

DNA is the basic element that controls all the processes that go on in the body's functioning systems. When it comes to your skin, everything that is not externally compromised or age related can be attributed to your genetics. Just as there are families with a genetic predisposition to cancer or diabetes, there are families with a conspicuous genetic bond when it comes to skin.

First, genetics determines the color of the skin: it determines whether you have light-colored skin or dark-colored skin. Genetics determines your amount of melanocytes, which are the pigment cells in the bottom layer of the epidermis, and how much melanin the melanocytes make. At one end of the spectrum are super-fair-skinned Celtics, who are at the highest risk for sun-induced skin cancers, and at the opposite end of the spectrum are African Americans. The darker the color of a person's skin, the more innate protection that person has against both the degenerative effects (lines, wrinkles, sunspots, broken capillaries) of the sun and the precancerous and subsequent cancer-causing effects of the sun, and therefore the fewer wrinkles and less skin cancer that person will have.

Some people have a genetic predisposition to skin cancer that is almost independent of ultraviolet irradiation. It's just in their DNA. And like melanoma, certain other skin conditions can be familial—such as basal-cell nevus syndrome, a genetic defect in which lots and lots of basal-cell carcinomas are present, or the rare BK mole syndrome, in which hundreds of precancerous moles (dysplastic nevi) develop into melanoma.

If you've got acne, chances are you have Mom and Dad to thank for it. Acne is predicated on oil production, and it's possible to inherit overactive oil glands. The causes of acne are based on oil production and the retention of dead cells within the lining of the pore or duct, both of which can have genetic susceptibilities, and therefore can be passed along from generation to generation. Nongenetically-related skin bacteria that live in the sebaceous follicle can also contribute to acne. These skin "bugs" can really aggravate your complexion.

There are also genetic ties to melasma and chloasma, specific discolorations of the skin discussed in chapter 1. An individual's sensitivity to the sun and his or her melanocytes' sensitivity to estrogen are based on heredity; the combination of these factors causes melasma or chloasma. But less specific discolorations induced by sun exposure are also impacted by genetics, since the lighter the skin color, the more sensitive it is to sun-induced tan and brown discolorations.

The bottom line on genetics' effect on skin is that genetics rules in making you susceptible to certain conditions, but alone is not a guarantee you will develop those conditions. Genetics merely makes you eligible. External factors and choices you make along the way feed in; genetics simply sets up the framework for what you're more or less susceptible to—in terms of your skin or any other organ.

The Sun

• • •

"Nature gives you the face you have when you are twenty.
Life shapes the face you have at thirty."

COCO CHANEL

Coco Chanel herself launched the sunbathing craze in the 1920s. She returned from a cruise with a deep, dark tan and single-handedly turned the tan into a fashion statement. I don't spend a lot of time in the sun, but I know that most people do—I see it every day on their faces. Those of you who have avoided exposing your skin to the wrath of the sun will have significantly better-looking skin than those of you who baked your bodies.

I don't tell my patients to stay out of the sun. Exposure to the sun is inevitable, but patients can learn to protect themselves from the damaging, harmful rays. Two simple solutions—wearing sunscreen and staying out of the sun at its midday strongest—will limit future damage, increasing skin's receptivity to restoring its collagen level (which makes skin suppler), and allowing skin to rejuvenate. Sun protection alone will never turn back the hands of time, but it will help to prevent future damage.

The sun has two different deleterious effects on the skin: degenerative and dangerous. Degenerative sun effects break things—they cause degeneration or harmless but unattractive distortions. The effects are not dangerous, but they are damaging and very annoying, especially if you want beautiful skin. The dangerous effects of the sun are precancerous and can go on to cause cancer when cells become sick. This malfunction becomes precancerous as a result of the ultraviolet radiation breaking DNA here and there in your skin and not having adequate means of repair. Those precancerous changes ultimately go on to become cancerous if not recognized and treated.

When the sun causes degenerative changes to the pigment cells, what is really happening is damage to the control mechanism by which the melanin cell (a melanocyte) makes melanin, causing it to make too much. When a melanin cell makes too much melanin, that

FACT: *Every hour, one American dies from melanoma.*

excess melanin feeds up through its dendrites to the overlying levels of the epidermis, causing a sun freckle, age freckle, liver spot, or solar lentigo. These are the most noticeable sun-induced pigment changes. (Light-skinned people tend to freckle more obviously.) These changes are generally not dangerous, though they are unattractive. Ultraviolet sun exposure can also cause small, irregular-shaped white spots, especially on the legs, but also on the backs of the hands and arms, as melanocytes are destroyed. The sun can also cause a malfunction in the exfoliation of cells. First the sun causes an excess of pigment, and next it causes the accumulation of cells that have pigment in them; the effect reinforces the depth or the concentration and intensity of the color of brown spots, making them darker.

UV radiation also causes the walls of blood vessels to become thinner, leading to bruising—with only minor trauma—in sun-exposed areas. For example, most of the bruising that occurs on sun-damaged skin occurs on the back of the hands and forearms—not on the inside of the upper arm or even the inside of the forearm. The sun also, by thinning the blood vessel walls, weakens them so they stretch and become engorged with more blood, making previously invisible blood vessels appear as conspicuous—but tiny—red squiggly or straight lines called *telangiectasias*. These tiny blood vessels occur in the skin, especially on the face.

The sun causes textural changes to the skin because UV exposure can cause a thickening of the upper layers of the epidermis and/or thinning of the lower layers of the epidermis and the entire dermis. Thick skin is found in coarse wrinkles—especially on the back of the neck—that do not disappear when the skin is stretched. This condition is called *solar elastosis* and is seen as thickened, coarse wrinkling and yellow discoloration of the skin. Thinning of the skin causes fine lines, wrinkles, easy bruising, and skin tearing.

An increased number of moles, especially junctional nevi, can form from brief but intense sun exposure (the type that causes blistering sunburns). They often progress to abnormal precancerous moles called dysplastic nevi. Other precancerous lesions, called *actinic keratoses,* are another possible effect of the damaging UV rays of the sun and are especially common on the face, ears, and back of the hands. They are small, rough, crusty, scaly red patches or sores on the top layer of the skin. Genetics and cumulative (rather than brief and intense) sun exposure are the main determinants for actinic keratoses. People

> FACT: *Actinic keratoses affect more than 10 million Americans, and in sunny climates their prevalence is significantly higher.*

with fair skin, light hair, and light-colored eyes are thought to be most sensitive and at risk. Those people with a history of extensive sun exposure and those who work or spend a lot of time outdoors have a greater chance of developing these spots. If left untreated, they can progress to an invasive type of skin cancer called squamous-cell carcinoma. *Seborrheic keratoses,* which are warty-looking lesions that appear to be stuck on the skin, are another common effect of the sun (although they can also be age related) but they do not become cancerous.

IN 2004, A TOTAL OF 7,910 *deaths were attributed to melanoma—5,050 men and 2,860 women. Older Caucasian men have the highest mortality rates from melanoma, and it is the chief cause of cancer death in women aged 25 to 29.*

The most dramatic, harmful, and life-threatening effect of the sun is *skin cancer.* The three main skin cancers are *melanoma, basal-cell carcinoma,* and *squamous-cell carcinoma.* Melanoma is the most deadly skin cancer because it metastasizes more readily and aggressively than the other skin cancers, and it is the metastases—the cancer's spreading to other parts of the body—which can result in death. Treatment of metastatic melanoma is very difficult. It usually arises from a pigment cell in a preexisting mole or from a previously normal single melancyte living peacefully in the basal epidermal layer.

Those most at risk from melanoma include the following:

- People with a large number of moles.
- People with red or fair hair, blue eyes, fair skin, and freckles.
- People who tan with difficulty and burn in the sun (Fitzpatrick skin types I and II).
- People with a family history of the disease. (For those who have already had melanoma, the chance of getting a second tumor is only increased by 11 percent.)
- People who have had blistering sunburns.

More women than men get melanomas, mainly in the thirty-to-sixty-year age group, but it can strike women or men at any age. However, children are rarely affected because even if they've had extensive exposure to the sun, it takes years for the melanoma to develop. When children do get melanoma, it is testimony to the importance of genetics in this disease. It is believed that 80 to 90 percent of our lifetime damaging exposure to the sun occurs by age twenty, and the amount of exposure during early years is actually one of the most important determining risk factors for melanoma—and for all skin cancers. Although melanomas can affect most parts of the body, it is most common for women to get them on the legs and arms, and for men to get them on the trunk, particularly on the back.

Melanomas can grow two ways: horizontally, giving rise to superficially spreading melanomas—less dangerous because they take longer to spread—or downward (nodular melanoma), causing the cancerous cells to invade blood vessels and lymph vessels earlier, so they spread sooner and kill faster. There's strong evidence that melanomas occur on sun-damaged skin and that people at the highest risk are those who have had sudden, very high intensity short bursts of sunlight in places where the sun is very strong.

Melanoma is one of the most unforgiving cancers. Once it spreads, it's almost always fatal. The only effective way to fight this killer is to prevent it.

On the other hand, basal-cell carcinoma, the most common skin cancer, grows and invades locally rather than metastasizing, so it is much more limited in the damage it can do and almost never kills. It develops in the basal layer of the skin—the same bottom layer of the epidermis where the melanocytes are. It is associated with aging and years of chronic sun exposure.

Squamous-cell carcinoma is the second most common skin cancer, which develops from the middle and outer layers of the epidermis. It is one of the forms of skin cancer closely associated with aging and years of sun exposure. It can metastasize and therefore be fatal, although not as commonly as melanoma. It is much more apt to metastasize if it occurs in sun-protected areas—the underarms or beneath bathing suit areas—or on mucous membranes such as the lips. Of course, it should be treated as soon as it is detected.

The risk of getting basal-cell carcinoma or squamous-cell carcinoma is determined by a person's lifetime exposure to UV radiation and by the person's pigment protection. Over the past sixty years, damage to the planet's ozone layer has increased the amount of harmful UV radiation that reaches skin.

The UV radiation that reaches the earth is made up of UVA and UVB rays. UVA rays age the skin and UVB rays burn the skin. Both can cause skin cancer. UV radiation is not felt as

(continued on page 74)

> **SKIN CANCER**
>
> *is the most common of all cancers, accounting for nearly half of all cancers in the United States. The incidence of skin cancer is rising dramatically, with more than 1 million new cases expected to be diagnosed this year.*

How You Can Help Prevent Skin Cancer

HOW TO EXAMINE YOUR BODY (monthly) for skin cancer, precancers, and abnormal moles:

1. Pick a well-lit room—preferably with natural sunlight. Examine yourself in the same place each month.

2. Examine your body front and back in the mirror; then examine your right and left sides with your arms raised.

3. Bend your elbows and look carefully at your forearms, upper underarms, and palms.

4. Look at the backs of your legs and at your feet, especially the spaces between the toes, and the soles of the feet.

5. Examine the back of both your neck and scalp with your hand mirror. Part your hair for a closer look. (Use a hair dryer on a cool setting to help part the hair.)

6. Finally, check your back, buttocks, and genitals with your hand mirror.

7. During the exam, look for these changes in all skin growths:

   - sudden or gradual increase in size
   - change in shape—especially concave borders, which are never normal
   - increased elevation (above the skin)
   - softening or hardening of the growth
   - itchiness, tenderness, or pain
   - bleeding, crusting, or oozing
   - redness, swelling, or new blemishes on the skin around a lesion.

If you notice anything suspicious or detect any of these warning signs, contact your dermatologist immediately for a professional evaluation as well as a full-body skin exam. Make sure to point out areas of concern and discuss them with your doctor.

ACTINIC KERATOSES AND SKIN CANCER

	APPEARANCE	SIZE	LOCATION
ACTINIC KERATOSES	Rough, scaly sandpaper patches, crusts or sores, typically pink to red	¼" to 1"	Face, scalp, neck, lower lips, ears, forearms, and back of hands
BASAL-CELL CARCINOMAS	Small, shiny bumps or nodules that are red, pink, or skin-colored; persistent nonhealing sores that crust and/or bleed; reddish flat patches or bumps with a central depression	Take many years to reach ½"	Head, neck, hands, and occasionally the trunk of the body
SQUAMOUS-CELL CARCINOMAS	Red, scaly patches, nodules or bumps; irregular shape; bleed and/or crust	Can reach up to ¾" to 1" or larger	Face, ears, scalp, neck, lips, back of hands, back, and legs
MELANOMAS	Asymmetrical, mottled patches with notched or blurred borders, typically in tan, brown, or black with multiple colors or hues and irregular colors and shapes	Can be as small as 1/16", rarely greater than an inch	Can occur anywhere on the body, most frequently on the upper back or legs, as well as on the head and neck

PROGRESSION	POTENTIAL FOR METASTASIS	PREVALENCE		
Most progress into squamous-cell carcinoma over a period of years	Are, by definition, precancers and therefore do not metastasize	Very common, affect more than 10 million Americans, especially Fitzpatrick types I and II	*Actinic keratoses, typical*	*Actinic keratoses, advanced*
Slowest-growing of the skin cancers—evolve over many years and may bleed, crust over, then repeat cycle	Very rare, but can grow into adjoining areas and may invade any adjacent or underlying structures including eyes, nose, etc.	Account for 80 percent of all skin cancers (more than 800,000 new cases each year)	*Basal-cell carcinoma, typical*	*Basal-cell carcinoma, advanced*
Can develop into large masses and invade underlying tissue or metastasize	Can metastasize and may be fatal if left untreated. When arising in sun-exposed areas, rarely metastasize; when arising in non-sun-exposed areas or on the lips they are much more aggressive and dangerous	Account for 16 percent of all skin cancers (about 200,000 new cases each year) with 2,200 deaths a year	*Squamous-cell carcinoma, early stage*	*Squamous-cell carcinoma, advanced*
May begin in or near a mole or other dark spot on the skin or, less commonly, appear without warning	Will metastasize if not removed at a very early stage; rarely cured after metastasis occurs	Account for 4 percent of all skin cancers (about 54,200 new cases each year) with more than 7,600 deaths a year	*Melanoma, early stage*	*Melanoma, advanced*

heat on the skin, so even on a cool and cloudy day, it can be just as strong and just as damaging as on a clear and sunny day. So you can still get burned on cloudy days and incur significant sun damage. Are you ready to put on some sunscreen yet?

If detected early, skin cancer has a 99 percent cure rate. To spot skin cancer early, you need to be vigilant in conducting self-examinations and making regular visits to your dermatologist. A recent study showed that people who regularly examined their skin for suspicious moles cut their risk of death from melanoma to nearly half that of those who did not do exams. Check yourself every month—like the wise women who do a monthly breast exam on themselves. You may think you get most of your sun exposure in the summer, but that doesn't mean you get no exposure the rest of the year. Also, skin cancer doesn't necessarily show up right away—so it's important to conduct body examinations monthly throughout the year. You'll want to be in a brightly lit room with a full-length mirror and your trusty hand mirror, too. Look for moles and other skin growths that display any of the potential signs of cancer: a new bump or spot; a sore that doesn't heal; an asymmetrical blemish; a notched, blurred border; a mixture of colors; or a diameter of at least six millimeters (about the size of a pencil eraser). Any change you can detect is not a subtle one but an important one and should immediately be shown to a dermatologist; by the time you can see a change, it's already significant.

Smoking

Everyone realizes that sun exposure is a risk factor for skin cancer, but almost no one knows that smoking is also an important and independent risk factor. Smoking more than triples the risk of developing squamous-cell carcinoma.

When it comes to your skin, smoking exposes you to the worst environmental poisons you can encounter. It has two effects on your skin: internal and external. Internally, smoking cuts down the circulation within the facial skin by 30 to 40 percent. Cutting down circulation cuts down the flow of nutrients necessary for repair of injury and for normal metabolism. Most people know that smoking is terrible when it comes to heart disease because it causes constriction of coronary vessels, but most aren't aware that smoking also causes constriction of skin blood vessels. That's what gives heavy smokers a sallow or pale appearance. The presence of the toxic chemicals causes constriction of the skin blood vessels and squeezing out of the blood—the resulting paleness is the opposite effect of the skin redness caused by the opening up of the skin's blood vessels from drinking alcohol.

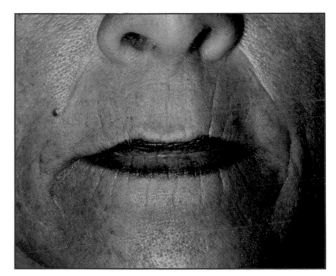

Smoker's lines.

It is really difficult to override the efficiency of the normal metabolic processes in the body and skin, but smoking is so damaging it does just that. As long as smokers continue smoking, their facial-skin color will be slightly off. When and if they stop, the color will come back.

Smoking's external effect on skin is caused by the chemical carcinogens and toxins from exhaled smoke. These carcinogens affect the skin from the outside in, promoting skin cancer.

Additionally, smokers use muscles in the lips that nonsmokers don't use as frequently. By virtue of overuse of those muscles and repetitive subjection of that skin to certain mechanical stresses, the elastic tissue and collagen break down, causing vertical lines that are often referred to as smoker's lines—on both the upper lip and the lower lip. I can tell a smoker just by looking at the distribution of these vertical lines, which are significantly out of proportion to other facial lines and to other signs of intrinsic or extrinsic aging.

Smoking's most perceptible effect on the skin is the causing of wrinkles—lots of them. Some reports suggest that smoking switches on a gene involved in destroying collagen, the structural protein that maintains the skin's normal thickness and contour. When you lose collagen, you get lines and wrinkles—not a great trade-off for smoking. Smoking has also been found to create dangerous free radicals. This results in oxygen deprivation to the

FACT: *The facial wrinkles of smokers aged 40 to 50 are similar to those of nonsmokers 20 years older.*

body's cells and reduces blood flow to the skin, which then causes premature wrinkling and sagging. Just ten minutes of cigarette smoking decreases the body's—and skin's—oxygen supply for almost an hour. Nicotine narrows blood vessels and prevents blood from circulating to the capillaries (tiny blood vessels) in the upper layer of the skin. The wrinkle effects are reversible if smokers quit early enough—but the lines and creases created after decades of smoking are impossible to reverse without laser surgery or filler injections three to four times a year.

And smoking's negative effects don't stop there. Another common side effect of smoking involves the hair. Did you know that smokers are three to six times more likely to develop premature thinning and graying of the hair? Smoking is even associated with causing ill effects on the circulatory system and on wound healing. It has long been known to interfere with patients' recovery from an array of surgical procedures. It takes a smoker a longer time to heal, and there is traditionally more scarring.

Human Nature

• • •

"Reality is a crutch for people who can't cope with drugs."

LILY TOMLIN

As long as our planet continues to exist, and our Western culture, values, and priorities remain, there will always be people in hot pursuit of becoming better looking. We live in a world where we only want what we don't have, not what we've got. So if we have beautiful eyes, we want fuller lips. If we have peaches-and-cream color, we want a smoother, more lustrous texture. It's human nature and it's an incredibly strong driving force in the demand for cosmetic dermatologic services. It's like that great line from the film *When Harry Met Sally*: "I want what she's having!" It's fun to fantasize about looking better—to transform ourselves into imaginary beings who live in a world where we have the features we think are

FACT: *Men who smoke are twice more likely to become bald than men who do not smoke.*

missing, the absence of which prevents (in our minds) certain successes in life, whether social or professional.

There's an old saying that goes, "If I had known I was going to live this long, I would have taken better care of myself." Touché! I saw a recent episode of the hit show *Nip/Tuck*—a show about two Miami-based plastic surgeons and the patients they treat. Joan Rivers was a guest on the season finale; she played herself. She went to these doctors and asked them to perform the ultimate plastic surgery: undo all the work she'd had done. She wanted to look like the woman from Larchmont, New York, who she would have been if she had never become famous. The surgeons were taken aback by her request, but considered the opportunity. After much deliberation, they showed Joan Rivers, via computer-generated graphics, what she would have looked like had she not had any of her plastic surgery or cosmetic dermatological procedures. It was a shocking revelation. Joan was virtually unrecognizable to herself. Needless to say, she was not nearly as appealing as she appears with all of the extra "help" she's had. Ultimately, she opted to *not* cosmetically turn back the clock she chose to stop years ago.

The basic human drive to look better, along with time, sun damage, bad choices, and genetics, dictates the demand for better skin. How many of us would have taken better care of our skin in our youth if we had known then what we know now? If you could have looked into a crystal ball when you were eighteen years old (slapping baby oil all over your body, using a metallic sun reflector to make sure you soaked up every ray of sun possible) and seen yourself at age sixty-five, seventy-five, and eighty-five, what would you have changed? If you could have gotten a preview of the degenerative effects of all your abuse, would you have done something different? Would you have worn sunscreen? Would you have taken better care of your skin? Would you have moisturized and sloughed off those dead cells more often?

My point is this: imagine being able to perform some kind of magic to erase your years of bad choices and to allow yourself to look better, feel better, and appear younger than you do right now—without plastic surgery. Well, let me tell you: you can have beautiful skin without magic. All you need to do is start making better choices, limit your external contributing factors, and take better care of your skin. Would you do that? If you said yes, the next chapter is the first day of the best skin you've ever imagined.

CHAPTER

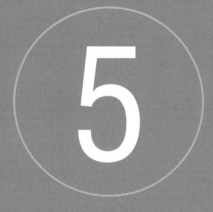

5

"*I listen with love to my body's messages.*"

LOUISE L. HAY

Diet and Skin

SKIN IS A GREAT MIRROR OF YOUR HEALTH. It can reflect good health, or conversely, illness. Think of it as an outside marker of what's happening on the inside. Nutritional deficiencies, diseases, and even stress may first be reflected in your skin's appearance.

Since skin is the largest organ of your body, it makes perfect sense that something interfering with your body could manifest itself in your skin, right? Think about it. Each square inch of your skin contains blood vessels, sweat glands, and nerve endings, which measure your body temperature, pain, touch, and pressure.

The skin has many vital protective functions: it protects the underlying tissues from invasion by bacteria, other microorganisms, the sun's harmful rays, and toxic substances in the environment. In addition to keeping undesirable things out, skin keeps moisture and needed chemicals in.

Like all organs in the body, the skin, as well as its appendages—like hair and nails—receives nutrition via the bloodstream from nutrients absorbed in the gastrointestinal tract. Believe it or not, the skin receives up to one-third of the blood circulating in the body! This illustrates perfectly why it is essential to nourish your skin from the inside.

Most *topical* nutrients and supplements we hear so much about these days, such as the proteins collagen and elastin, essential oils, and most vitamins simply cannot be absorbed into the cells of your skin. There are some topical medications, such as cortisone-type creams, alpha hydroxy acids, and a derivative of vitamin A called retinoic acid that are exceptions, but for the most part, the best method of nourishing your skin is making careful choices about what you put into your mouth. The foods you eat can make a meaningful difference when it comes to the appearance of your skin.

VITAMINS AND MINERALS THAT HELP YOUR COMPLEXION

As I've said before, it is extremely difficult to override the normal metabolic processes of the body. When I hear about schemes and empty promises that suggest you take more of this vitamin or more of that mineral, I cringe at the millions and millions of dollars people spend on false hopes. You can take thirty pounds of a vitamin and it won't do a thing for you if it isn't what your body needs. It's like pushing harder on a light switch to make a room brighter. Either the switch is on or it's off. That's exactly how it is when it comes to vitamins, which are really special enzymes, and your body. Extra amounts of an enzyme do nothing to change the rate of chemical reaction.

I am going to make an assumption that most of you are pretty well nourished and that you're basically getting the right amount of vitamins and minerals in your daily diet. You are getting enough iron, vitamin A, B, C, and D, and essential amino acids—all the *essential* (meaning you can't manufacture them yourself, you have to eat them) elements it takes to run the metabolic machine of the human body. And if for some reason you are not eating the right foods, you are hopefully supplementing your mild deficiencies. The important thing is to understand what foods you should include in your daily diet to be certain you are getting all of the essential vitamins and minerals to help keep your skin looking and feeling great.

For example, your body converts **beta-carotene** into **vitamin A,** so eating a healthy dose of beta-carotene every day helps generate new skin cells and can even help protect against skin cancer. Foods such as apricots, peaches, nectarines, sweet potatoes, tomatoes, spinach, and carrots are all great sources of beta-carotene. Although vitamin A deficiencies are rare in industrialized countries, certain digestive diseases or excessive gastrointestinal surgery can result in impaired absorption of this vitamin. Vitamin A deficiencies lead to reduced sebum production, clogged hair follicles, and excess keratin buildup, giving the skin a dry, rough, and scaly appearance. Please note, however, that if your facial skin *is* dry, rough, or scaly, it probably does *not* mean you have a vitamin A deficiency; it's simply worth noting the possibility.

Vitamin C is essential in building new collagen; citrus fruits, berries, melon, tomatoes, papaya, spinach, and sweet potatoes are good sources of vitamin C. A vitamin C deficiency can bring on all sorts of problems, but the most common is scurvy, which affects the skin and is characterized by poor wound healing, small purplish spots called petechiae—indicating bleeding below the surface of the skin—ulcers, and gum weakness. Scurvy can also cause excess keratin in hair follicles, producing roughened bumps containing coiled hairs on the arms and legs.

Selenium, which is an antioxidant found in fish, garlic, chicken, and grains, works with *vitamin E* against pollutants, sunburn, and even skin cancer. Selenium helps maintain the quality of the skin. It functions internally to help close wounds.

Since **vitamin E** is hard to get from food without eating too much fat, the best sources are oil-rich nuts, seeds, and avocados. Recent studies demonstrate that as much as one-fourth of topical vitamin E use causes a rash called contact dermatitis. I firmly believe vitamin E is essential in the diet to maintain healthy-looking skin, but I do not support any purported topical benefits.

Calcium is important for preventing sagging skin and wrinkles. The best sources of calcium are broccoli, spinach, tofu, salmon, and soy products. Dairy products, although well touted as good sources of calcium, are not the best choice. Our digestive system simply can't break down dairy products and absorb their calcium so that it is of any use to our system. You're better off taking a calcium-enriched vitamin or even a daily dose of Tums Calcium to properly absorb your daily calcium.

Niacin (one of the members of the vitamin B complex) deficiencies can cause a condition called pellagra, which is characterized by rough, scaly brown skin in areas of the body exposed to the sun—especially the neck and upper chest. It's uncommon today, except among alcoholics, some cancer patients going through chemotherapy, and people who take a number of drugs—including certain antibiotics, anticonvulsants, and antidepressants—that can interfere with niacin metabolism. Niacin can be absorbed through lean meats, poultry and fish, peanuts, rice bran, and dairy products.

Likewise, a **riboflavin** deficiency can adversely impact skin, causing scaly, greasy red skin around the nose and mouth and on the ears and eyelids. Sebaceous material builds up in the hair follicles, giving the skin a roughened look. The lips can also become red and cracked from a riboflavin deficiency. Many nonsugary, fortified breakfast cereals contain riboflavin.

A deficiency of **biotin** produces scaling skin. Uncooked egg whites contain a substance that prevents absorption of biotin. So for all of you egg-white lovers, make sure eggs are thoroughly cooked. You can supplement biotin in your diet by eating liver, unpolished rice, brewer's yeast, whole grains, sardines, and legumes.

Those of you on low-fat diets may not be getting all of the **essential fatty acids** your body needs to avoid scaly skin and even hair loss (something very near and dear to this doctor's heart, not to mention my head). If you are on a low-fat diet, make sure to supplement with *linoleic acid,* which is found in vegetable oils; it can correct this deficiency. Another concern I have in this world of fad dieting are low-protein diets, which can cause a condition known as kwashiorkor, seen mostly in children in underdeveloped countries, but not rare in this country. It is characterized by dry, wrinkly, flaky skin; thinning hair; and a loss of hair color. The protein deficiency produces scaly skin, and the loss of skin protein through excessive scaling aggravates the deficiency. Children are especially at risk and must eat a balanced diet consisting of some protein (a serving of fish, chicken, or meat) at least once a day to avoid this condition.

Men and women who suffer from an **iron** deficiency will notice the early sign of brittle nails with a flattened spoon shape. This often precedes the pale skin associated with iron-deficient anemia. Cracks may develop at the corners of the mouth, and hair growth may be affected. An iron deficiency can be detected through a simple blood test, long before symptoms of anemia set in. Make sure you check with your doctor if you notice any of the above signs.

Finally, a severe **zinc** deficiency results in widespread blisters and peeling skin lesions—especially in skin creases and on the fingertips. In less extreme cases, the signs can be more subtle, such as dry skin, a scaly scalp, and slight hair loss.

Because vitamin deficiencies are proven to have harmful effects on the skin, it might seem to make sense that taking vitamin supplements would help in achieving or maintaining healthy skin. While I don't think vitamins necessarily Influence a positive effect on skin for those eating a balanced diet, an overload of certain vitamins can most certainly adversely affect skin. Excess vitamin A, for example, results in cracked lips and dry, scaly, itching skin. Excess beta-carotene can produce a generalized yellowing of the skin, especially the palm and soles, almost simulating jaundice. Excess niacin may cause chronic itching, facial flushing, and warmth. Too much vitamin E can cause an allergic rash, and overdoses of vitamin D may result in intense itching.

Another thing to avoid in your diet, besides overdoing your vitamin intake, is overdoing your **alcohol** intake. Aside from the obvious pain of the day-after hangover, chronic alcohol use has damaging effects on virtually every organ system, especially facial skin. Have you ever noticed how puffy and sallow your skin looks after a night of heavy drinking? Alcohol dehydrates your skin (and the rest of your body) and causes small blood vessels to dilate and widen, allowing more blood to flow close to the skin's surface. This causes puffiness under the eyelids and an overall bloated appearance. This also produces a flushed skin color and a feeling of warmth, but actually decreases body temperature as your body heat escapes from the excess blood in these engorged blood vessels.

Another effect of drinking alcohol is "blood sludging," in which the red blood cells clump together, causing the small blood vessels to plug up, starve the tissues of oxygen, and cause cell death. With this increased pressure and the direct dilating effect of alcohol on the skin vessels, capillaries break, creating the red, blotchy skin seen on heavy drinkers' faces. This also prompts a lowered resistance to infection, since alcohol depresses the immune system.

A weekend of celebration involving too much alcohol may cause a breakout in people who are acne prone or who suffer from rosacea. However, such an occurrence is predictable and preventable for those people if they avoid overdoing it.

Alcohol prematurely ages the skin because it dehydrates it, robbing precious moisture and often significantly worsening skin conditions such as psoriasis. Research indicates that women who average two drinks a day, four days a week, are more than twice as likely to develop melanoma as women who don't drink. For good health and the sake of a beautiful complexion, alcohol consumption should be as limited as possible. Experts recommend that women limit themselves to one drink a day, and men—who also get skin cancer—to two drinks a day.

The right diet may slow down skin aging, but the reality is it won't stop it. The more vegetables, legumes, fish, olive oil, and low-fat dairy products people eat, the healthier their skin looks. Some studies have even shown that people who eat a healthier diet are prone to fewer wrinkles than those who eat more meat, sugar, butter, and whole-milk dairy products. Eating a diet high in fat may also promote the development of basal- and squamous-cell carcinomas. Although avoiding excessive sun exposure is still the best way to avoid skin cancer, it now appears that eating a low-fat diet may be a good second line of defense.

As early as 1939, animal studies indicated that among mice, those fed a high-fat diet and exposed to ultraviolet radiation developed cancer at higher rates than those on low-fat diets. There's significant evidence today that shows humans react much the same as the mice. A recent study by researchers at Baylor College of Medicine in Houston found that eating a high-fat diet promotes the development of premalignant tumors and skin cancers associated with UV exposure.

The bottom line is, to prevent increasing your chances of skin cancer, use more sunscreen and eat less fat.

The ultimate key to healthy skin and nutrition is to be aware of your needs. Talk to your doctor about what vitamins and/or minerals you are lacking and the best way to supplement your diet.

> FACT: *People who eat a high-fat diet are five times more likely to have one or more actinic keratoses—premalignant lesions—than people who eat a low-fat diet.*

SOME FALLACIES ABOUT SKIN AND NUTRITION

My patients tell me all sorts of crazy stories that they hear from friends or read in the paper or on the Internet about nutrition and its effect on skin. So how do you know what to believe?

It's simple: Chocolate does not cause acne. Neither does fried food. Oily foods do not influence the skin's degree of oiliness—only male hormones can increase the activity of oil glands. And unless you are allergic, or suffer from rosacea, spicy foods and nuts do not cause redness of the face. (Certain foods, such as cayenne pepper, tomatoes, alcohol, and even coffee affect rosacea sufferers, triggering flare-ups when consumed.)

Food allergies and skin rashes have been linked for many years—hives caused by food allergies come from a variety of foods like shellfish, nuts, and many fruits—but the connection between the two is greatly overemphasized. Generally, if you have suffered from food allergies, your most important piece of evidence linking a certain food to a skin problem is your own history of outbreak. In addition to resulting from eating certain foods, allergic skin reactions can come from *handling* foods; certain chemicals used to preserve food can make the skin more sensitive to sunlight. The best treatment for a proven food allergy is to eliminate the food from your diet. Same goes for contact reactions to food. It's like that old joke about the patient who comes into the doctor's office and says, "Doctor, it hurts when I go like this," waving his hand in the air. The doctor says, "So, stop going like this," waving back. If a food is adversely impacting your skin, stop eating or handling it.

There is one mineral found in food that adversely affects everybody's skin, allergy or no, and that's iodine. Iodine has a cumulative effect, so it causes acne breakouts—but only after a certain amount has accumulated over a period of weeks or months. Iodine in our systems comes from eating shellfish, lobster, shrimp, and crabmeat; certain greens from the ocean such as seaweed or kelp; or spinach. A seventeen-year-old teenage girl who has acne and is dieting, eating four spinach salads a week, is going to be adversely affected by iodine. She's simply getting too much iodine, preventing her acne from clearing up.

Another myth floating around is that your skin can absorb vitamins and minerals from cosmetics, to keep it from aging. Because the outermost layer of the skin is composed of dead cells, topically applied nutrient-based cosmetics don't have any long-term impact on aging. You simply can't feed the dead outer layer of skin to replenish minerals, protein, and vitamins. However, topical vitamin C in a stabilized preparation can be effectively absorbed in the upper layers of the skin, as an antioxidant helping to prevent sun damage. Newer

BEFORE: Demonstrating acne, reds, and large pores. The acne is best seen on her chin and cheeks, the diffuse red on most of her face from her lips up, and the large pores are best seen on her left cheek (right side of photo).

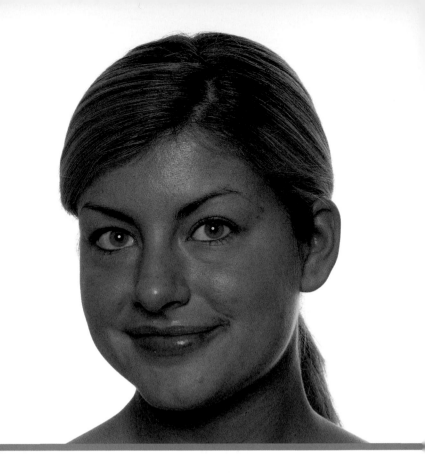

AFTER: Shows marked reduction in redness, pore size, and acne—a very good example of luster, and skin that is smoother and brighter. She's a very pretty woman who, in this picture, could be a model.

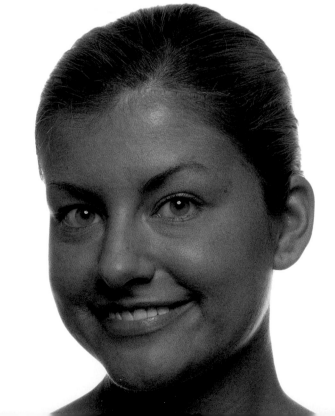

technologies are emerging which help topically applied chemicals penetrate into the skin where they can be effective—but this technology has yet to be perfected.

Collagen gets a lot of attention for supposedly being a great rejuvenator of the skin, and when injected, it's fabulous. But when applied to the outer layer of the skin, the collagen molecules simply cannot penetrate through the epidermis to the important second layer, the dermis, where it is needed. They bind water to the stratum corneum, the outermost layer of the epidermis, which may plump the skin temporarily, making it look and feel younger, but the effect is short-lived. Topically applied, collagen can help function as an effective moisturizer, but for that purpose it would be absurdly expensive.

Oil-based products, such as petroleum jelly, cocoa butter, and mineral oil contain lanolin, a fat derived from the oil glands of sheep. While lanolin helps the skin retain moisture, people with oily skin who use these products are actually doing more harm than good. By now you already know that adding oil to oil clogs the pores and can cause inflammation and irritation. Your skin surface may appear to be smoother and some fine lines and wrinkles might appear to fill out from using these products, but none of these preparations can stop aging of the skin. The topical application of certain minerals may change the skin's chemical or physiological activity, but that comes from a drug, not a cosmetic.

One final thought about diet and the skin. I've talked about an aging face as being partly dependent on the loss of fat. But, notice how people who are overweight tend to have fewer furrows and wrinkles in their facial skin. That's because they have a surplus of fat stored everywhere—including in their faces. But what happens if they lose that excess weight? There is an adverse effect on the appearance of the face. When you lose weight, you lose it everywhere—and for most people, the face is an indicator of weight gain and loss. So when you diet, you lose some of the protective effect of the extra adipose tissue in your face. This pre-diet fat fills out lines and furrows, much the same way collagen and certain fillers do. When you lose weight and decrease that layer of fat, you increase the appearance of lines, wrinkles, and even furrows. While this may be disappointing, I still advise losing the weight. Get your body healthy first and foremost. When you look better you feel better, and personal health is number one. Once you're back into your skinny jeans, I promise, a few extra lines on your face won't bother you. And, if they do, make sure you read chapter 11 to familiarize yourself with all your options, or see your dermatologist about filling those lines. Don't get me wrong—I'm not against fixing wrinkles!

CHAPTER

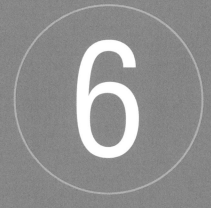

6

"The choices we make are ultimately our responsibility."

ELEANOR ROOSEVELT

Recapture and Restore Your Beautiful Skin

SKIN CARE FOR OUR GRANDPARENTS was a bar of soap, a splash of water, and maybe a little moisturizer. Needless to say, skin care has come a long way. The beauty industry churns out more than a thousand new products every year. In 2004 Americans spent almost $2.4 billion on over-the-counter products such as cleansers, antiaging lotions, and sunscreens. That number increases by another $5.3 billion if you add in bath additives, men's products, and powders.

We live in a society where, for many of us, looking younger and feeling healthier is a daily pursuit. According to the American Academy of Dermatology, the quest for younger-looking, softer-feeling skin translates into the average American female adult using at least seven skin-care products a day.

I'm the first to tell you that you absolutely do need some kind of skin-care regimen for your face, but using too many products that are not congruent, or that serve no additional purpose, is simply a waste of your time and money—two of the most important commodities in life. In some cases, you may be doing more damage to your skin if you are using the wrong products for your skin type and/or condition.

So how do you decide on skin-care products that are right for you?

The first step is determining your skin type. If you haven't already done so, refer to chapter 3. In review, there are six skin types: normal, oily/acne-prone, dry, combination, mature, and sensitive. Most of you will fall into one of the first five. Very few people actually have sensitive skin. The pivotal distinction concerning skin type is whether or not you have excessive oil production, because that is what determines whether or not you can use products that contain oil. People who have oily/acne-prone or combination skin must use products that are water based, oil free, or noncomedogenic. By the same token, people with very dry skin should not use a cleanser that extracts excessive amounts of water. Skin type can change with time, so it's important to stay in touch with your facial skin. You may need to adjust your products depending on the season—what's just right in warm, humid weather may be too strong or harsh in cold, dry weather.

The second step to choosing the right products for your skin is deciding what you want those products to do. Are you trying to fix your color? Texture? Both? Are you cleansing the skin, moisturizing, or protecting it? You can't choose the right product if you don't understand what you want it to do.

LET'S TAKE A CLOSER LOOK AT SOME COMMON PRODUCTS

Cleansers

A cleanser is any product that removes sebum (skin oils), dirt, and other undesirable substances from the skin. Cleansers range from very moisturizing to very drying and should be chosen to match your skin type. Any cleanser that acts through a process of emulsification will do the trick. *Emulsification* is the term used when the product contains a chemical that is able to grab oils off your skin by virtue of combining them with water, enabling it to bind and therefore remove oil, dirt trapped in the oil, and other debris. It doesn't really matter what's in the product, although I don't recommend perfumed soaps—the perfume serves no real function and can only cause potential irritations.

Bottom line: When it comes to choosing a cleanser or soap, keep it simple. If you find your skin becoming drier in the winter months, look for a milder soap that is fragrance free. In fact, many soaps today contain moisturizing ingredients like oils and vitamins, which can be beneficial for your skin all year round—unless you have oily skin. It is perfectly fine to use the same brand of soap throughout the year as long as your skin is not adversely impacted during the drier winter months.

CLEANSERS AND THEIR APPROXIMATE PROPERTIES

SOAPS AND CLEANSERS	MOISTURIZATION	IDEAL SKIN TYPE
Lipid cleanser	Very moisturizing	Dry, sensitive
Surfactant with oil	Mildly moisturizing	Moderately dry, mature
Surfactant with oil-free moisturizing ingredients	Neutral	Normal
Plain surfactant and acne cleansers	Drying	Oily

The simplest cleansers are oils and water. Normally oil and water don't mix, but cleansers or soaps create a bond between the oil and water in order to function as a detergent. Sebum and other oily materials will dissolve in oil. However, some dirt and debris substances will not dissolve in oil. Plain warm water will remove many of these substances, so the combination of rinsing with water and using oil is effective for cleaning the skin.

A lot of cosmetic companies market lipid cleansers because they are very effective in removing oily makeup. These cleansers leave an oily residue and are especially effective on dry skin. They are also gentle and effective for mature or sensitive skin. However, highly alkaline soaps and detergents are extremely drying and should be avoided. Many products on the market these days allege that exfoliation is the key to radiant skin. With dry or sensitive skin, however, it is crucial to remember that mechanical exfoliation by harsh abrasive ingredients such as fruit pits or sea salt strips the skin of any natural barrier it has built up, and can cause extreme dryness and irritation. With dry or sensitive skin, any exfoliation must be chemical (using an alpha- or beta hydroxy acid) and very gentle. The most important thing when choosing a product for these skin types is to look for the gentlest formula available.

Water-free oil products are the most moisturizing by virtue of their ability to enhance water retention, whereas water-based products can only add moisture without necessarily effectively retaining it. Please note, water-free products may induce acne and should be avoided for oily and acne-prone or combination skin; they won't leave oily skin feeling clean. When someone with oily skin, acne, or even combination skin uses a soap with oil in it, like Dove—which is terrific and the cleanser I recommend for dry or sensitive skin—their condition can get worse. When someone with sensitive skin uses a soap such as Ivory—allegedly one of the purest soaps known to humankind but sometimes moderately irritating—their skin can become aggravated. On the other hand, a soap like Ivory is very effective as a cleanser for oily/acne-prone skin.

Now I am going to share a very tightly held secret of mine: I wash my face with plain soap and water. I have done so for nearly thirty years. I have oily skin, so for me, I find plain soap (I use Ivory) and water works very well. Interestingly, Ivory soap is advertised to be $99\frac{44}{100}$% pure. Because of its purity, it's marketed as one of the safest and best soaps to use on babies. Despite its purity, its extremely effective and strong oil-emulsifying and removal properties make it much more useful for teenagers with acne (and this dermatologist) than for babies' bottoms.

Soaps are surfactants, which are salts derived from plant and animal oils or fats. Soap-free cleansers are detergent cleansers that are synthetic and contain no soap. Surfactant cleansers, which are soaps, soap-free cleansers, and soap/detergent combinations, can be made with added oil to make what is probably a mildly moisturizing product for moderately dry skin. Alternatively, they can be made with added oil-free moisturizing ingredients such as humectants, esters, or fatty acids; these are sometimes referred to as superfatted soaps. These products are relatively neutral and are perfect for normal skin. Some superfatted soaps claim to be for dry skin; however, there are better choices for very dry and mature skin. Plain surfactant cleansers are somewhat drying because they remove oil from the skin without replacing it and are therefore best for oilier skin.

I'm often asked about the irritancy of soaps, which can be a relatively controversial subject. Many people believe that plain soap is not good to use for cleansing your face. I disagree. I think that using the right soap for your skin type is the most important thing—even if it's simple. The purpose of soap is to get unwanted debris and dirt off your skin. You can go really no-frills and simple when choosing a cleanser as long as it works for your skin type.

The normal skin pH is a range between 5.6 and 5.8, the latter of which is slightly acidic. The least irritating cleansers have a basic pH but can be irritating when left on the skin for extended periods of time. In contrast, most soap-free cleansers and soap/detergent combinations have been modified chemically to have a lower pH so that they will be less intrinsically irritating. If soap is rinsed thoroughly from the skin after use, chances of irritation are significantly reduced. It's important to wash off as much residue as possible, noting that some soaps rinse off more easily than others. One of the functions of using a toner/astringent after washing is in fact to remove any cleanser residue.

Acne cleansers can be surfactants with the addition of therapeutic agents or exfoliating agents common in acne medications—such as benzoyl peroxide, sulfur,

ACCORDING TO THE FINN CHAMBER TEST, which measures irritancy of soap and cleansers by leaving them on the skin for lengths of time far exceeding normal washing, the following list denotes the relative irritancy of some of the most commonly used soaps (least irritating to most irritating):

1. *Dove*
2. *Aveeno*
3. *Alpha Keri, Dial, Fels-Naptha, Neutrogena, Purpose*
4. *Ivory, Jergens, Lowila, Lubriderm, Oilatum*
5. *Basis, Cuticura*
6. *Irish Spring*
7. *Camay, Lava, Zest*

or salicylic acid. Alternatively they may be drying solutions of alcohol or witch hazel, which really puts them more into the category of toner/astringent. Abrasive scrubs that contain particulate matter are sometimes marketed "for unplugging the skin pores" in acne. Many abrasive scrubs extol the benefits of removing dead surface skin cells; however, it is debatable whether some of these scrubs actually do more harm than good by creating inflammation or by paradoxically thickening the skin from overuse and overzealous harsh scrubbing. Aluminum oxide and ground fruit pits or nut shells are supposedly more abrasive than polyethylene beads, which are in turn more abrasive than sodium tetraborate decahydrate granules. I recommend ground-fruit-pit or nut-shell scrubs for the body, but not for the face. If you have severe acne, overzealous use of an abrasive cleanser will be too harsh for your already irritated skin and may worsen your condition. What all this means is that you have to read the label of the products you are considering carefully. With all topical skin-care products, less is more and gentle is always better than overzealous.

In my opinion, dead surface cells should be removed with chemical exfoliants that gently dissolve the dead cells, and the real benefit of abrasive or particle scrubs is in their ability to unplug skin pores with gentle use at the end of a shower (when the pores have been steamed open). A gentle fifteen to twenty second massage with your fingertips on the large-pored areas will enable the scrub's particles to dislodge the oil and debris that constitute the clogs in the pores, and which contribute to the appearance of large pores.

TAKING THE CONFUSION OUT OF SKIN CARE

I think what confuses most people about skin-care products is putting together a skin-care regimen using generic (nonprescription, store-bought name brand or store brand) over-the-counter cleansers, astringents, exfoliators, and moisturizers—and predicting whether they will work in harmony. There are advantages, therefore, of using one line of products specially or professionally formulated. For example, when recommending my own skin-care products, I know that the products have been patient proven and have demonstrated that they work harmoniously, without being too strong or too weak.

There must be a convergence and synergy of products in their respective categories to achieve success in your skin-care plan. You don't have to use my products to achieve your desired results, but you do need to select products that are synergistic—meaning they are designed to work well together and they are appropriate for your skin type. It's helpful to use proven, tried-and-true products to avoid any wild-card results and to stack the deck to ensure the results you want and need.

Toners

The cleansing process is really a two-step process. After using a soap or cleanser, the next step is to use a toner to remove any additional residual oil, dirt, or cleanser from the skin's surface. *Toner, clarifying lotion, freshener,* and *astringent* are really different names for the same thing. The purpose of toner is to dissolve things off your skin, not to put anything on. Despite claims to the contrary, none of these products will make your oil glands produce less oil, nor will they permanently shrink your pores. The most they will do Is make pores appear smaller by causing a temporary swelling, tightening, or slight irritation.

Most toners basically consist of water, alcohol, fragrance, and in some cases, coloring. Alcohol-free toners are made for sensitive, very dry, and mature skin. In addition to high levels of alcohol, products for oily skin generally contain astringent ingredients such as witch hazel and menthol. Some might also contain resorcinol, which acts as a combination antiseptic, preservative, and astringent, and whlch may help to remove dead surface cells.

Toners complete the cleansing process by removing any leftover debris, oil, cells, or cleanser so that your skin is evenly and consistently cleansed. The two-step cleansing and toning process not only prepares the facial skin to allow the active ingredients in corrective products to perform in an optimum fashion, but it also enhances their ability to fix what is broken—that is, to improve your color and texture. For some people, soap and water alone does the trick; however, for most of us, that is simply not enough to thoroughly clean the surface of facial skin.

In order for a cleanser to accomplish this two-step process by itself, it would have to be very strong and would probably cause irritation. Using a gentler cleanser plus a toner creates a certain predictability; it optimizes the efficacy of and reduces the possibility of irritation from products—and contributes gently and safely toward removing impurities that need to be eliminated. And the best way to ensure predictable and consistent results from active ingredients is to strip off all of the excess oil, impurities, dirt, debris, and dead cells on the skin.

Remember, every product you use should be predicated on your skin type—and toner is no exception. Toners for normal skin usually contain mild cleansing ingredients as well as other ingredients that soothe the skin and aid in moisture retention. These products may contain variable levels of alcohol, rose water, castor oil, glycerin, sodium borate, and allantoin.

Toners for dry, mature, and sensitive skin include very mild cleansers and skin-soothing ingredients. They contain no alcohol and are most effective at making the skin feel refreshed. People with dry skin or eczema should avoid toners that contain high levels of alcohol, salicylic acid, or resorcinol, since all these ingredients can dry out already dry skin, making the condition worse instead of better.

Toners for oily and combination skin are formulated to help remove more oil and therefore often contain more alcohol. This can leave oily and (especially) combination skin somewhat dry, particularly on the cheeks, and so may require the use of a water-based moisturizer on any dry areas to compensate for the overdrying.

Now that you can identify your skin's defects and your skin type, you'll be able to read the labels on skin-care products to ensure that you are buying products that are right for your skin and that will not make it worse. Manufacturers are now motivated to label skin-care products as water-based, oil-free, or noncomedogenic, because there has been an increase in consumer demand for this information—which is critical to choosing products for oily, acne-prone, or combination skin. Now you know to read labels carefully as you move forward in your pursuit of recapturing and restoring your skin's health and beauty.

Cleansers and toners are the two products being shouted from the rooftops by skin-care companies, but it's important to note that this one-two combination is not enough to see changes to your skin's color and texture. To do this, you must use an active ingredient.

Choosing an Active Ingredient That's Right for You

The outer layer of the skin consists of dead cells that are constantly being sloughed off and replaced. The sloughing process, when it works properly, reduces and helps eliminate discolorations and textural issues, resulting in a complexion that is more radiant, youthful, and healthy looking. Unfortunately, the sloughing process doesn't always work as it should. By your late twenties or early thirties, skin that has not had the benefit of some kind of exfoliation is dull looking, often discolored, and less vibrant. As skin ages, dead-cell sloughing naturally slows down and doesn't work properly, causing the accumulation of undesirable dead cells. But not to worry—cosmetic manufacturers have developed numerous products to aid this natural sloughing process. Products that help remove the dead cells, normalizing the process, are called exfoliators.

Normal skin needs the least amount of help in sloughing off dead cells, since it does it quite adequately by itself. Removing the outer layers of cells from the epidermis, especially if the skin is rough, makes light reflect more evenly and improves the overall appearance of the skin. For an exfoliator to really work, it requires at least one active ingredient. The active ingredient is what acts as an exfoliant.

Exfoliating can be mechanically accomplished through such procedures as microdermabrasion or shaving and scalpel abrasions, or through the use of products that incorporate granules into a cleanser or cream. Or it can be chemically accomplished through active ingredients such as alpha hydroxy acid (glycolic acid, lactic acid) or beta hydroxy acid (salicylic acid).

Salicylic acid is found in dozens of over-the-counter products, and when used in small doses and at low concentrations, can be mildly effective over time without being irritating—as it is in higher concentrations. Salicylic acid has been used for many years as a peeling agent for the skin. It's commonly found in astringents, cleansers, and creams for dry, flaky skin, aging skin, and acne. While it is helpful in removing dead cells in low concentrations, it can't accomplish what other chemicals can, by virtue of its irritancy when used at higher strengths. It is excellent for helping treat common ailments such as razor bumps from shaving, rough and/or dry skin, as well as mild acne, and it can help to reduce mildly uneven pigmentation such as freckles and age spots.

One of the great skin-related buzzwords and therapeutic successes of the last decade has been AHA, or alpha hydroxy acid. Alpha hydroxy acid is only slightly different in chemical structure from salicylic acid, which is a beta hydroxy acid, or BHA. But when scientists discovered alpha hydroxy acids and their utility, they used the term *AHA* in a mysterious way, as if they had invented something groundbreaking. Consumers didn't realize the close similarity of AHA to salicyclic acid, so they immediately started replacing old salicylic acid products with new AHA products. Both are pervasive in over-the-counter products and are used to remove dead cells for fixing brown and tan color as well as dull texture. AHA products are much more effective than salicylic acid products for color and texture skin problems.

Alpha hydroxy acids are a group of naturally occurring acids derived from certain plants, fruits, and natural products, including sugarcane, apples, grapes, citrus fruits, sour milk, and rice. History suggests these "fruit acids" have been used for hundreds of years as moisturizers and skin fresheners. Ladies of the French court and women of ancient Rome used aged wine, which contained tartaric acid, to improve their skin. Over the last ten years, medical research has advanced our understanding of these AHAs and allowed us to create better formulations of these products. We now use AHAs to combat acne and dull, weathered, sun-damaged skin, and to fix many of the color and textural problems that prevent beautiful skin. AHAs can also help reduce fine and medium facial wrinkles.

AHAs work by dissolving the "glue" that holds dead cells together on the surface of the skin. This allows the dead cells to slough off, leaving behind a layer of smoother, and thereby brighter and softer, skin. In addition, AHAs help to dissolve the material that clogs pores. This allows the pore to drain better, decreasing the tendency for the formation of acne lesions and helping to reduce pore size and the appearance of enlarged pores.

The problem with salicylic acid is that while it works, it's not really effective enough in the concentration available in over-the-counter products. AHAs, on the other hand, have really created a revolution in our ability to correct skin color and texture. AHAs are a family of chemicals, the three most common of which are lactic acid, glycolic acid, and pyruvic acid.

The first AHA used for skin care was derived from lactic acid, and was introduced in the mid-1970s by Westwood Pharmaceuticals as ammonium lactate; it is still available as a product called Lac-Hydrin. Sold in weaker strengths in over-the-counter products, and in stronger strengths by prescription only, it is mostly used as a body moisturizer that further acts to remove superficial, scaly dead cells. The moisturizer is reasonably good and the small amount of lactic acid does help to chemically dissolve some of the dry scales. It's interesting to note that Cleopatra took milk baths for the purposes of restoring her skin; milk contains lactic acid, which makes the skin smoother by removing dead cells.

But for the purposes of skin repair and restoration, the most useful AHA is glycolic acid. Glycolic acid is a very simple, small molecule made from the chemical manipulation of sugar and sugarcane. Glycolic acid is much stronger than lactic acid, and much more keratolytic—meaning it dissolves keratin, which the uppermost dead layer of the epidermis is made of. For that reason, it is the optimal chemical agent for restoring even color and smooth, bright texture to the skin.

All acids have different strengths. They can be concentrated, or they can be diluted to be very weak. A lot of over-the-counter products claim to contain glycolic acid, but most have so little in them that they just can't possibly be effective. Worse still, some products are labeled with words that look or sound like *glycolic,* but contain no glycolic acid and so offer none of its benefits. The bottom line: The strength of glycolic acid is critical to its effect.

I believe glycolic acid is the most effective active ingredient—with the widest therapeutic margin—of all the keratolytics. You have to use it in the right strength and form to see results. Most over-the-counter products with glycolic acid don't go much above 3 or 4 percent in content, meaning they won't be as effective as physician-strength glycolic acid products. *Physician-strength* implies higher strength. "Lunchtime" glycolic peels done in a physician's office have become very popular because they offer much greater benefits than glycolic products used at home (although physician-strength home products, when used properly, are still quite effective). This procedure removes just enough of the top layer of dead skin cells to leave skin looking rosy and radiant, but allows you to immediately go back to work as if you had no procedure at all. The benefits are wonderful and visible after just one or two treatments.

Finally, pyruvic acid, another AHA, is much too strong for use by consumers. A doctor may use a pyruvic acid in the office to do a controlled peel of the skin, but it certainly wouldn't be a superficial peel, like glycolic acids peels are. A pyruvic acid peel would remove enough layers of the skin to cause crusting.

In my opinion, the three therapeutic active ingredients mentioned so far, salicylic, lactic, and glycolic acids, as well as cleansers and toners, are all safe for use during pregnancy when used as directed. However, a pregnant woman should always consult her obstetrician before putting any topical agent on her skin.

On the other hand, one product that should never be used by pregnant women is tretinoin, which is also known by the brand names Retin A, Avita, and Renova. These products have been shown to be teratogenic in rodents—meaning they cause malformations in rodents' developing fetuses. Retin A, a brand of tretinoin, was very popular in the late 1970s and early 1980s, and was used primarily for the treatment of acne. It was later discovered to have a positive effect on photoaging by reducing fine lines, and it became the first topical chemical for reducing fine lines at home. It was also shown to help reduce brown spots.

Retin A, Avita, and Renova have a very narrow therapeutic margin, and some patients are very easily irritated by the products. Tretinoin is also photosensitizing, so it's much easier to get sunburned when using it. Finally, tretinoin can cause neovascularization, or the production of tiny blood vessels, and can break capillaries, causing red color issues instead of erasing them. Renova, which is tretinoin in an emollient base, was developed for an older, non-acne-prone population. It has a heavier and more moisturizing base because older people have drier, less oily (mature) skin. Renova was patented for the purposes of fighting photoaging, or to help reduce fine lines. Women come into my office all the time asking for Renova, but in my experience it is not nearly as effective and certainly much more difficult to use than glycolic acid for the treatment of color, texture, and (some) contour problems.

In summary, although alpha- and beta hydroxy acids have been described by some doctors as being old news, I believe they are and will remain state-of-the-art, essential fixtures in effective skin care and dermatological practices.

Sunscreens and Moisturizers

The final products you need to complete your skin-care routine are a sunscreen and a moisturizer. Let's look first at the importance of using a sunscreen.

The application of sunscreen should be done 365 days a year. The concept of protecting your skin from future damage is predicated on taking steps to ensure your skin's safety. Whether I like to hear about it or not, there are many people who enjoy the warmth of the sun on their skin; it feels good. We all participate in outdoor activities, whether jogging in the morning, walking to work, taking the kids to school, eating at an outdoor café, or walking the dog. It's simply unrealistic for me to tell patients to stay out of the sun completely. If I did, they'd either find a new dermatologist or they simply wouldn't listen. Hopefully the sun will shine for many more millions of years, and therefore the best advice I can offer is to tell you how to protect yourself when you are outdoors.

Sunscreen helps prevent sun damage, both degenerative and precancerous, including brown spots, broken capillaries, wrinkles, and actual cancers. Sunscreen, like every facial product you use, should be predicated on your facial skin type.

Most sunscreens are moisturizers with added sunscreen ingredients. There are also oil-free emulsions, solutions, and gels available especially for those of you with oily or acne-prone skin. It is extremely important to use a sunscreen that is right for your skin type.

Sunscreens display their SPF (sun protection factor) on the product label. The SPF indicates the amount of UVB light that will pass through the product when applied in a layer of standard thickness. It also tells you how long the product allows you to stay out in the sun without burning in relation to how long you could stay out without burning if you weren't wearing sunscreen. A sunscreen with an SPF of 15 will allow one-fifteenth of the UVB light striking it to pass through to the skin.

Let's say you live on the East Coast, and it is noon on a beautiful, eighty-degree, bright, sunny day in mid-July. Without sunscreen, if you have type I or II skin, you will develop a sunburn within fifteen minutes. If you use a sunscreen with an SPF of 10, in theory, you can stay out ten times longer, meaning one hundred fifty minutes (two and a half hours) before you will burn. But SPFs are a little like EPA ratings. When you look at the EPA rating on a

> FACT: *More than $1.2 billion was spent on moisturizers last year.*

RECOMMENDED SUNSCREENS FOR VARIOUS SKIN TYPES

SUNSCREEN TYPE	IDEAL SKIN TYPE	BASE TYPE	FORM
"Waterproof" Note: No sunscreen is really waterproof	Dry, normal, mature	Oil based or absorption	Stick, oil, ointment
Water resistant	Dry, normal, mature	Water in oil	Cream, lotion
Regular	Normal to dry, mature	Oil in water	Cream, lotion, spray
Oil free	Oily, acne prone, combination	Oil free or water or alcohol based	Cream, lotion, spray, or gel

new car, there's always a disclaimer stating that you may not get the same mileage posted on the sticker on the open road, because mileage with respect to gas economy is determined under laboratory conditions, as are SPFs.

A good rule of thumb is that all SPFs shrink by one-third in actual use. When sunscreen is tested, it is tested in a lab with no wind, no spray of water, and less perspiration. So a sunscreen with an SPF of 15 really shrinks to an SPF of 10 in actual use. I always recommend using a sunscreen with an SPF of at least 15 to 30. A sunscreen with an SPF of 15 gives you 88 percent protection from sun damage caused by UVB sunlight. A sunscreen with an SPF of 30 gives you 95 percent protection. If you double the SPF from 30 to 60, you only gain another 4 percent in protection (99 percent). I don't know that the last 4 percent is worth it, considering how unpleasant, thick, and gooey many sunscreens with an SPF of 45 to 60 tend to be—although they can be more acceptable to people with mature skin. For women, an alternative to wearing sunscreen (which I only recommend when you don't have access to it) is to wear makeup with an SPF number. Foundation, lipstick, and moisturizers with an SPF of 8 or higher are common.

I think the SPF-number system has confused some consumers. In the near future, the FDA is expected to change the requirement for SPF numbers, so that sunscreen manufacturers

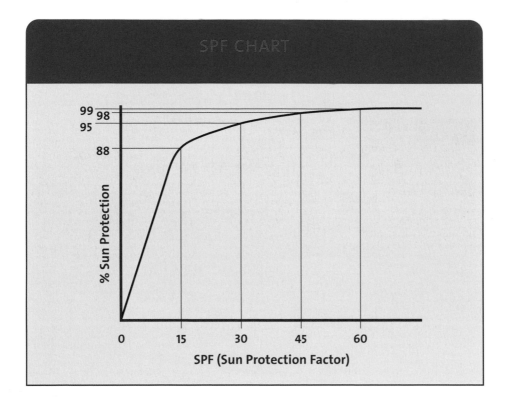

SPF CHART

% Sun Protection (y-axis): 88, 95, 98, 99

SPF (Sun Protection Factor) (x-axis): 0, 15, 30, 45, 60

will no longer have to put numbers on their packaging; they will simply label their product as low, medium, or high protection.

It used to be said that sunscreen shouldn't be used on infants under six months of age, but recent studies have shown sunscreen to be harmless to their young, beautiful, soft skin. But all things considered, I still recommend keeping babies six months and younger out of the sun—period.

In addition to sunscreen, you need a moisturizer to keep your skin in balance. Moisturizers are designed to add moisture to the skin—whereas emollients are designed to soften the skin. However, adding moisture to the skin tends to soften the skin, and therefore the terms *moisturizer* and *emollient* tend to be used interchangeably. If the stratum corneum (outer layer of skin) contains less than 10 percent water, the skin feels dry. Surface oil plays an important part in preserving dry skin by acting as a barrier that prevents evaporative water loss. Therefore, traditional moisturizing products are oil-concentrating products. The more oil a moisturizer contains, the more effective the moisturizer becomes, but the greasier and

EFFECTS OF MOISTURIZERS ON VARIOUS SKIN TYPES

TYPE OF SKIN	MOISTURIZER BASE TYPE	NET EFFECT
Extremely dry or mature	Oil based	Extremely moist
Very dry or mature	Absorption	Very moist
Dry	Water-in-oil emulsion	Moderately moist
Normal to dry	Oil-in-water emulsion	Mildly moist
Normal to oily	Oil free, water based	Slightly moist

(to some people) the more unpleasant it feels—and the more apt it is to aggravate acne in people with oily and combination skin.

Finding the right moisturizer is an integral part of any skin-care regimen. One way to improve even the best moisturizer is to apply it when the skin is still damp, because what a moisturizer does, essentially, is lock water on the surface. Your skin (especially dry skin) needs its water (moisture) replenished; this is what moisturizers are supposed to do. Oil glands can't compensate for the lack of moisture: oil is not a substitute for water. Water-based, not oil-based, moisturizers increase the water content on the outer layers of the skin, and give it a softer, more comfortable feel. An oil-based moisturizer is really an "oil-izer" that works by holding in or retaining existing moisture. But if there is no moisture to hold in, it can't function effectively as a moisturizer.

Cleanser, toner, an active ingredient, sunscreen, and moisturizer are the products you will use in your daily program. It is essential to find the right products that work harmoniously for your skin type and condition. For more help figuring out which products are right for you, see chapter 8. There you'll find a complete list of conditions and recommended products.

DRY-SKIN TIP

Use a cold-water humidifier to add moisture to your environment, especially when you sleep and in the winter. This will help to reduce the amount of moisture lost from the skin through evaporation.

CHAPTER

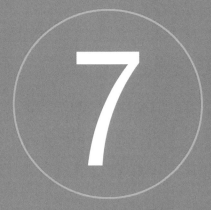

7

*"If we take care of the minutes,
the years will take care of themselves."*

BENJAMIN FRANKLIN

The Program

WHENEVER I'M ASKED WHY I DEVELOPED my own line of skin-care products, I always respond "because my patients needed them." Perhaps like you, my patients don't always understand how to choose products that will work for their skin and their conditions. Most patients come into my office with some degree of color and texture issues, and they simply can't separate them from their contour (lines, wrinkles, jowls, furrows) issues. So I developed my own line of products revolving around my notion that patients know they're unhappy when they look into the mirror, but they don't know what they're unhappy with. If you can't identify the problem, how can you effectively treat it?

If you've ever used the computer program Photoshop, you know that an image is made up of a composite of several layers superimposed on each other, each layer with a different element that makes the final picture. But unless you have an understanding of that program and its effective use of superimposed layers, you can't possibly decipher all the elements making up the final photo. The same holds true for your facial skin: when you look into a mirror, you are looking at a composite of several different layers that make up your facial skin and ultimately your outward appearance. And unless you are a dermatologist, you probably don't yet understand those layers' implications on your overall appearance. But my products, and the program laid out here, were developed to take the guesswork out of skin care.

Every condition on your face falls into one of three categories: color, texture, or contour. The combinations and permutations of the elements that compose these three categories cause dissatisfactory reflections. So when my patients have that inevitable "aha" moment, when they finally make the connection between their skin and their condition, my products make sense to them. I can show them how to use the products that are right for their skin, products developed especially for those color and texture issues, and they understand the issues and ask for the right products. They ask for something to lighten their brown spots or to take away their dead cells. They get it. And so will you.

ACHIEVING PERFECT SKIN

In addition to a perfect skin-care program, getting enough sleep, eating a healthy, nutritious diet, and finding adequate relaxation time all positively impact having the skin you've always wanted.

There are endless products available that can address your skin-care needs, but the most important issue is to use the right products for your skin type and for your specific concerns. I promise: if you follow this very simple program, consisting of understanding the three categories of your skin (color, texture, and contour) and then using products appropriate for your problems and your skin type, you will see a rapid and noticeable improvement in your complexion's color and texture within fifteen to thirty days.

The program doesn't take a lot of effort. In fact, it doesn't even require you to use my products. However, it does require you to be diligent and consistent. It takes two minutes to do, but isn't your skin worth two minutes twice a day? The bottom line is, no product works in the bottle; it only works on the face. The program is almost foolproof in its simplicity. When used as prescribed, it works for almost everyone.

THE SIMPLE FOUR-STEP PROGRAM

This program leads you down a clear path so that you can achieve the beautiful, healthy skin you have always wanted. My simple technique makes better-looking, healthier skin achievable for everyone—as long as they follow the plan. There is no excuse for a dull, tired, dry, patchy, blotchy, discolored-looking complexion. Not anymore.

Look, skin care isn't like ordering from a Chinese take-out menu. You can't choose one item from column A and another from column B and expect the products to work in sync. Products are designed *together* to work effectively *together*. I deliberately planned my skin-care line to complement the ultimate goal in improving color, texture, and contour.

But before you get started on your new regimen, let's review the steps you've already taken. In chapter 1, you learned to identify those defects that make up the various problems on your face, including color issues such as red and brown spots and texture issues such as dry, flaky skin; dull-looking, matte, tired skin; and acne-prone, large-pored, and cobblestone skin—and you marked them on the face diagram you filled out in chapter 1.

You've identified the areas that need improvement, and you've (hopefully) accurately ascertained your skin type, in chapter 3. Identifying your correct skin type is crucial to finding the right products to improve the quality and appearance of your skin. In chapter 6 you read about the five main products you need to correctly recapture and restore your bright, radiant, glowing skin—a cleanser, a toner, an active ingredient, a sunscreen (for day), and a moisturizer (for night). Finding the correct products for your skin should be far less daunting than it used to be now that you know exactly which products to look for.

My program breaks down your routine into a morning regimen and an evening regimen. The first three steps are exactly the same for both. You will cleanse your skin, use a toner, and then use an active ingredient. Your morning routine will then include a sunscreen, your final product before applying makeup. The difference in your evening routine will be using moisturizer as your fourth and final product. Using sunscreen and moisturizer on a daily basis will help prevent your problem from coming back or worsening and will help maintain a normal balance of water and oil in your skin.

To make it easy for you to follow, I have broken down the morning and evening routines into two separate sections.

MORNING ROUTINE

Step One: Cleanse the Skin

In order for an active ingredient to work, we all need to start from an even playing field. That means removing oil and debris that will prevent an active ingredient from penetrating the skin. Everyone, regardless of skin type, has to prepare their face to accept any topical treatment by using a cleanser and a toner appropriate for their skin type.

Cleanser begins the preparation process. Never vigorously scrub your face or use a washcloth; applying excessive pressure to an already inflamed, chafed, or sensitive area will only make it worse. The cleansing process should be gentle: use your fingertips to massage a small amount of cleanser onto your face for ten to fifteen seconds, and rinse with warm—not hot or cold—water.

Step Two: Prepare the Skin with Toner

Toner completes the cleansing process by removing any leftover debris, oil, cells, or cleanser, so that you start with the same skin surface every time you wash your face. Apply toner to a soft, thin cotton makeup pad and gently wipe to remove any excess debris.

Now the facial skin is prepared to allow the active ingredients in corrective products to perform in an optimum fashion.

Step Three: Use an Active Ingredient

The next step is choosing and using the right active ingredient for your skin-care issues—in the appropriate form (solution, serum, cream, lotion, or ointment) for your skin type. If the active ingredient is not in the right form, it will be ineffective, or worse, may aggravate your problem.

The vehicle, or form, depends on your skin type. While every one of my products is labeled according to skin type, not all skin-care products make it that easy for you.

Many skin-care producers instead label products for oily, acne-prone, or combination skin as "water based," "oil free," or "noncomedogenic." The product need only use one of these terms—you don't get extra results or efficacy from a product labeled with two or all three, so don't waste your time looking. If you have dry skin, make sure that water is one of the first ingredients listed. If you have mature skin, oil or oil-based ingredients should lead the ingredient list, and water should appear somewhere later on the list, since your skin thirsts for both. If you really have sensitive skin, you'll be very lucky if you find products labeled "for sensitive skin," so you will probably have to resort to the ingredient list. Most important, make sure there's nothing in the bottle that will irritate your skin (such as salicylic acid). And if you have normal skin—lucky you! Most of us do, and therefore most products not labeled as being for the other five skin types will be just fine to use.

WHEN USING MORE THAN ONE ACTIVE INGREDIENT, *begin with the product that is in the lightest form. Use water- or alcohol-based products first; solutions, serums, or lotions second; creams third; and petroleum-based products last. A lighter product will never penetrate a heavier product.*

Sometimes you will need to use more than one active ingredient; the synergistic mechanism of two or more active ingredients can often increase efficacy and results. For example, for brown discolorations, after cleansing and toning the face, first use a bleaching product, which stops the skin from making additional brown pigment. Second, use an exfoliant, such as a glycolic-acid product, which removes extra pigment that already exists in dead cells. The continued use of glycolic acid will help prevent the accumulation of dead cells, which contributes to brown discolorations *and* to dull, matte skin. Furthermore, it will remove some of the early abnormal cells, which might otherwise go on to become precancers.

Glycolic acid is the most effective active ingredient in treating brown color and texture defects—but more is not always better. It must be started at the proper strength, which for most patients is 8 percent. The strength can slowly be advanced to 10 percent and ultimately 15 percent to optimize improvement. Advancing the strength is only suitable provided no irritation occurs during use. Most people without sensitive skin can easily ascend to the optimal efficacy of 15 percent—over a period of time.

Step Four: Apply Sunscreen

After using the active ingredients, which ameliorate the problem, the next step is applying sunscreen. Use sunscreen in the morning after the first three steps, but before applying makeup. Reapply as needed during the day if you spend a lot of time outdoors, work out, or perspire. Review chapter 6 to help determine the correct sunscreen for your skin type.

BEFORE: Her chin shows acne and brown spots of post-inflammatory hyperpigmentation from the pimples and from picking, as well as some redness from areas where pimples were and the skin is healing. Similar discoloration of reds and browns are evident on the upper lip. On the cheeks, next to the nose, her pores are slightly increased in size.

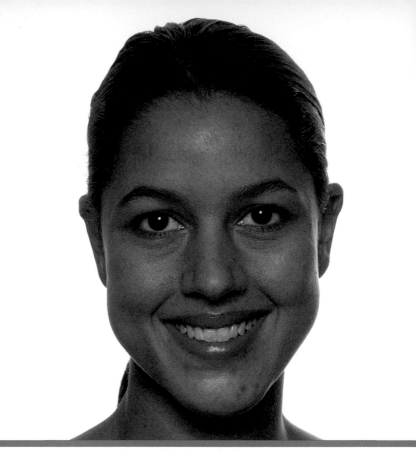

AFTER: Marked improvement in red and brown discolorations as well as in her acne. Illustrates luster and brightness (without an oily sheen) as a result of improvement in both the texture and the oil/water balance of the skin.

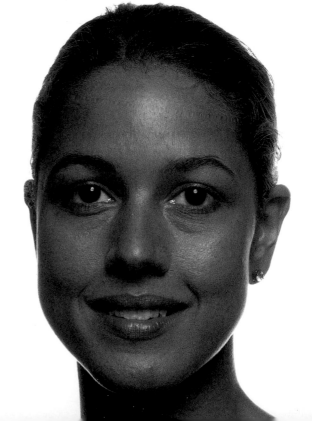

EVENING ROUTINE

Step One: Cleanse the Skin

(as described in your morning routine)

Step Two: Prepare the Skin with Toner

(as described in your morning routine)

Step Three: Use an Active Ingredient

(as described in your morning routine)

Step Four: Apply Moisturizer

In the evening, the final step is applying moisturizer. Be sure to use the right moisturizer for your skin type. Refer to chapter 6 for a detailed recap on choosing your correct moisturizer.

Using sunscreen and moisturizer on a daily basis will help prevent your problems from coming back or worsening and will help maintain a normal balance of water and oil in your skin.

> TIP: *Take a photo of yourself before you begin the program. Take another photo thirty days later. You will be amazed at the changes in your facial skin!*

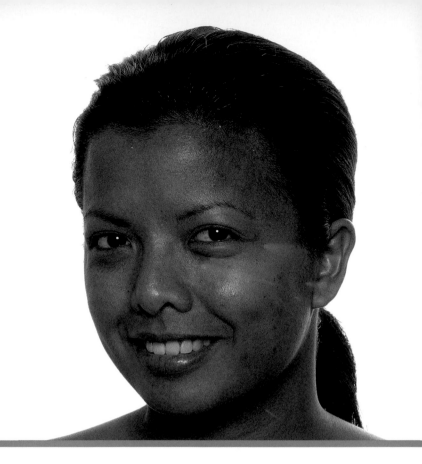

BEFORE: Shows acne, brown spots, blotches, and large pores. The discreet brown spots on her cheeks are post-inflammatory hyperpigmentation as a result of prior acne lesions (pimples and cysts). Active acne papules can be seen above her left eyebrow (right side of picture). The very dark small spot just next to her nose is a normal mole (junctional nevus is the technical name).

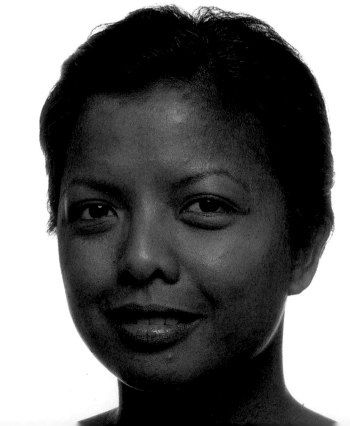

AFTER: Demonstrates decrease in brown spots, including the area above her lip, improvement in acne bumps, and decrease in pore size. As expected, the dark spot (normal mole) next to her nose is unchanged despite improvement of the other brown issues. (Mole color is unaffected by the program.)

If you are truly motivated to get the most out of this book and this plan, and if you truly want to optimize the appearance of your skin, you have to be prepared to make this process a daily practice. From this point forward, it's all about maintenance—both in getting to your desired results and in maintaining them. Just as you get up every morning and brush your teeth or comb your hair, take two extra minutes to practice the simple techniques I've shared with you. Think of it like successful dieting. Most people who go on diets lose weight, but put it right back on—and then some. The only way people keep weight off is by changing their eating habits and routine—their lifestyle. They stay on a particular plan to maintain their weight loss, which requires daily maintenance. It's all about discipline. Discipline in any routine results in success. And it only takes four minutes a day!

It is possible to recapture and restore your youthful, bright, radiant skin. It's not only possible, it's incredibly easy because you now understand what you're looking at when you examine your face. You can identify your problems, you know your correct skin type, and you have the simple technique to not only choose the appropriate skin-care products for your problems but to practice daily maintenance to preserve your beautiful skin.

The earliest signs that the program is working should start within the first two weeks. Subtle changes occur in color and texture that are noticeable to you through touch. You will notice your makeup goes on easier and smoother and that it takes less to cover imperfections. Another wonderful benefit of the program is that other people will compliment you as if you've done something—have you recently taken a vacation or changed your hair? They won't be able to pinpoint exactly what is different, but they will certainly want to know your secret! Once you've been on the program thirty days or more, you will not only feel the difference in your skin, you will be able to actually see the differences in your color, texture, and even contour.

Your success is predicated on your commitment and motivation—and by now, by virtue of you getting this far in the book, I know you're ready to put your best face forward.

CHAPTER

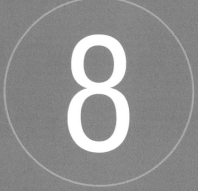

8

"You only get what you give yourself—so give yourself the best."

DR. ROBERT ANTHONY

Skin Type–specific Products for Your Program

YOU MIGHT THINK THAT IT HAS NEVER BEEN EASIER to choose the correct products for your skin type, right? Well, I'm not so sure. I had an eye-opening experience as I walked down the skin-care aisle of a major national drugstore. I was absolutely shocked, even confused, by the dizzying array of skin-care products on the shelves—and I am a professional skin-care authority! It is easy to understand why people are completely baffled, disempowered, and—ultimately—paralyzed in their ability to choose skin-care products, as a result of the incredibly large and intimidating selection. Without the help of the information contained in this book, without an understanding of their skin type and problems, how can anyone possibly make the right choices?

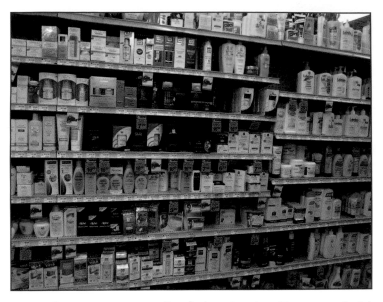

No wonder consumers are confused when choosing skin-care products!

Products in the skin-care aisle I visited were grouped by brand name, not by skin type or condition. Within the grouping by brand name, there was no particular consistency, no easy way to identify which products were cleansers, which were toners, which were active ingredients for pimples or facial rejuvenation, or which were sunscreens. And within the same brand, there were competing but similar products with only very subtle differences between them, which required the wisdom of Solomon and the expertise of a cosmetic dermatologist to decipher.

Neutrogena products were the easiest to figure out because in general they were clearly marked for each of the six skin types discussed in this book, but there were *sixty-two* Neutrogena products to choose from! There were also thirty-five L'Oréal products, forty-nine Olay products, sixteen Aveeno products, and twenty-eight Clean & Clear products, not to mention house-brand products and at least fifteen other brands.

One of my hobbies for the past twenty-five years has been studying, collecting, and of course, drinking wine. When I first started, walking into a wine store was even more confusing than my recent visit to the skin-care aisle was. But now I can visit any wine purveyor and walk up and down any aisle, and virtually every bottle will make some sense to me in terms of the type of wine, the vintage year, the grapes, the wine maker or winery, the country of origin, and the region of origin. Yet most people who have not studied wine find that walking up and down wine aisles can be as or more confusing than walking up and down skin-care aisles.

Best Cellars is a national chain of wine stores that has tried to simplify the selection and purchase of wine for regular consumers whose desire to drink and enjoy wine exceeds their technical understanding of it—by separating all of their wines into categories that consumers can more easily identify with. Those categories are: fizzy (obviously, champagnes and sparkling wines), fresh, soft, luscious, juicy, smooth, big, and sweet. Each category has a sign under which are a variety of ten or fifteen wines, which fit into those respective categories and make it easy for non-experienced wine drinkers to buy a wine that suits their taste.

So my goal in this book is to simplify choosing skin-care products that will suit your color and texture problems—based on your skin type. You can fight your way through the skin-care aisle once you know your skin type, understand the category of product you are seeking for your problem (cleanser, toner, active ingredient, sunscreen, or moisturizer), and have the ability to read labels. Product labels are so important. However, they can also be confusing and even misleading, as they are sometimes purposefully written to make you think that they can do things they can't or that they have ingredients they don't.

For instance, many products are labeled alpha- and beta hydroxy but in fact don't have therapeutic alpha hydroxy acids or beta hydroxy acids. But they make you think that they do.

This brings me full circle to the reason I created the Stallex for Perfect Skin skin-care line. I now appreciate more than ever its value to my patients, because they don't have to go through the research, bewilderment, and guesswork of obtaining the right products. I have assembled products that work harmoniously to accomplish the laid-out goals, products that are very simply labeled according to skin type and therapeutic application, or the skin-care goal you want to accomplish.

Now that you have a more complete understanding of skin type, you have a better ability to discern and ascertain what combinations are right for you. The appropriate products—from cleansers to active ingredients—will effectively and efficiently solve your color problems (whether they're focal and just random spots, or diffuse and blotchy areas) and your texture problems (dull, tired, flaky skin or large-pored skin). In an effort to help you pick the right products as you wade through the skin-care aisle at your local drugstore, I have put together a comprehensive guide of products that can work together to give you the results you seek. I hope that this will help you make more informed choices so that you will be successful in your new skin-care program. All products are formulated for your specific skin type. These are recommendations—I know that these products work.

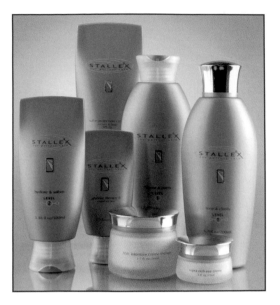

CHOOSING YOUR PRODUCTS

I have developed two of my own skin-care lines, Stallex for Perfect Skin—which I have included in the list of product choices—and Proof Skin Care. I have also chosen mainstream, easy-to-find skin-care products that will accomplish specific goals for various skin types. The bottom line is that you don't *need* to buy my products to accomplish your goal of being happy with your skin; there is a huge variety of products on the market that will allow you, in a cost-effective and easily accessible fashion, to choose cleansers and toners that will properly prepare your skin for other products that will improve it.

Many of these over-the-counter cleansers and toners are marked or labeled as to skin type. So it makes sense to buy products labeled "for normal skin" if you have normal skin, and "for dry skin" if you have dry skin. But products may not be labeled as being for mature skin; those labeled as being for dry skin can be substituted, for the most part. Conspicuous labeling can overwhelmingly be found on products for oily or combination skin. They are labeled as either "water based," "oil free," or "noncomedogenic," in addition to their being labeled for "oily," "acne-prone," or "combination" skin.

This guide is meant to help you find the right products for your skin and skin-related problems, but the real test of whether a product is right for your skin is how it feels after application. If a cream or lotion leaves your skin feeling irritated, it isn't working well for your skin.

If it leaves your skin feeling not too dry and not too oily, pleasant and in balance, then it's right for your skin.

For the most part, product ingredients are listed on product labels according to concentration. The product that is present in the largest percentage or proportion is the first item listed in the ingredient deck, or list. Each successive ingredient is therefore present in a lesser amount. This holds true until you get to the very, very low concentration ingredients—ingredients that make up less than 1 percent of the total product. At this point, the ordering is no longer by concentration, but these ingredients are usually preservatives and other stabilizers and are used for technical reasons. They don't usually have any significant relevance when it comes to your purposes for using the product.

So let's say you have oily skin, and the first ingredient in a product you pick up is mineral oil or petrolatum: chances are it's not for your skin. In fact, even if you have dry skin that is in need of moisturizing, you want to make sure that the first ingredient is water—not oil—because you want a moisturizer, not an oil-izer. On the other hand, if you have mature skin (lacking in both water and oil), then you do want a product with a high concentration of different types of oils or hydrocarbon-based chemicals.

So how do I know this program will work? I have had the opportunity to perform what is probably the longest and largest clinical skin-care study in the history of dermatology. For more than twenty years, I have seen tens of thousands of patients succeed using this program—using five or more accurately chosen products (a cleanser, a toner, one or more actives—which contain active ingredients—a moisturizer, and a sunscreen) that changed their skin forever. It worked for them, and I know it'll work for you. All you have to do is use the products.

• • •

SKIN-CARE PROGRAM FOR OILY/ACNE-PRONE SKIN

Acne. Pimples. Zits. Nine out of ten teens (and one out of five adults aged twenty-five to forty-four) suffer from these annoying, sometimes painful red bumps. Not to mention whiteheads and blackheads. A buildup of oil, bacteria, and dead skin cells can clog pores and cause acne. Stallex professional products and the following over-the-counter products can help you get long-term relief from this often embarrassing and now completely controllable condition.

Cleansers for Mild Acne:

Put your best face forward by keeping your skin fresh, clean, and clear. These facial cleansers cleanse normal to oily skin, and help you achieve and maintain a clear and radiant complexion.

Directions: Use two times daily and as needed to cleanse and remove excess oiliness. Gently massage with fingertips for fifteen to thirty seconds. Rinse with warm (not hot or cold) water. Pat, do not rub dry.

- *Aveeno Cleansing Bar for Acne:* 2% sulfur, 2% salicylic acid

- *Clearasil Medicated Deep Cleanser:* 0.5% salicylic acid

- *Fostex Acne Cleansing Bar:* 2% salicylic acid

- *Johnson and Johnson Clean & Clear:* alpha hydroxy, salicylic acid

- *Neutrogena Oil-Free Acne Wash:* 2% salicylic acid

- *Stallex Cleanse and Purify, Level 2:* our specialized ingredients dissolve and wash away dirt and oil from the pores to reveal your skin's clarity while maintaining its natural moisture.

Cleansers for Moderate or Severe Acne:

These antibacterial and anticomedonal facial cleansers for very oily and acne-prone skin work gently but effectively and help you maintain a clear and radiant complexion. Regular use will help control acne and prevent breakouts.

Directions: Use two times daily and as needed to cleanse and remove excess oiliness. Gently massage with fingertips for fifteen to thirty seconds. Rinse with warm (not hot or cold) water. Pat, do not rub dry.

- *Fostex 10% BPO Acne Medication Bar:* 10% benzoyl peroxide

- *Oxy-10 Daily Face Wash:* 10% benzoyl peroxide

- *Peter Thomas Roth Medicated BPO 10% Acne Wash*

- *Stallex Cleanse and Purify, Level 3:* formulated with 10% benzoyl peroxide, our cleanser penetrates deeply, dissolving oil and dirt to unclog pores and clear up blemishes.

- *Stallex Pore Minimizer Cleansing Grains*

Toners for Oily/Acne-prone Skin:

A toner completes the cleansing process by removing residual dirt, oils, dead cells, and cleanser. Skin is left feeling fresh, clean, and healthy.

Directions: Wash, then pat dry. Sparingly apply toner to a thin cotton pad and gently wipe affected area. As the residual oils and cells are extracted from the skin, the pad picks up a faint hue of yellow or gray. Repeat with fresh pad until there is no color change on pad.

- *Clearasil Medicated Astringent:* 0.5% salicylic acid

- *Clinique Oil Controller*

- *Neutrogena Antiseptic Cleanser:* benzethonium chloride, witch hazel

- *Stallex Tone and Clarify, Level 2* or *Stallex Tone and Clarify, Level 3:* these high-potency facial toners for oily or acne-prone skin gently and effectively cleanse and tone for fresh, clean skin all day long.

Active Products for Oily/Acne-prone Skin:

Regular use helps to prevent acne breakouts and reduce the appearance of enlarged pores. Each of these products has been formulated for facial rejuvenation and management, and prevention of acne in oily/acne-prone skin. Each also helps result in smoother, brighter, younger-looking skin, with improved texture and color.

Directions: Cleanse face and pat dry. Apply very sparingly with fingertips, using only two or three drops for entire face. Distribute evenly until fully absorbed.

- *Aqua Glycolic Astringent:* alcohol and 2.5% glycolic acid

- *Alpha Hydrox Oil-Free Facial Gel:* 8% glycolic acid

- *Glytone Day Cream for Oily Skin:* 10% glycolic acid

- *NeoStrata Oily Skin Solution, AHA 8:* 8% glycolic acid

- *Neutrogena Healthy Skin Face Lotion:* 8% glycolic acid

- *Peter Thomas Roth Glycolic Acid 10% Clarifying Gel*

- *Stallex Clear Control Solution*

- *Stallex Glycolic Therapy 15 Gel for Face and Body:* a concentrated high-potency gel formula for more aggressive revitalization, smoothing, and softening.

On-the-spot Treatments for Acne:

Antibacterial lotions fight acne breakouts. These products get deep into the pores, fight infection, dissolve oil, reduce inflammation, and promote healing.

Directions: Cleanse skin morning and night, then apply a very small amount to acne blemishes.

- *Clean & Clear Persa-Gel:* 10% benzoyl peroxide cream

- *Oxy Deep Pore Acne Medicated Cleansing Pads, Maximum Strength:* 2% salicylic acid

- *Neutrogena On-the-Spot Acne Treatment:* 2.5% benzoyl peroxide cream

- *Stallex Z Lotion:* combines effective acne-fighting ingredients with the added benefits of tea tree oil.

Moisturizers for Oily/Acne-prone Skin:

Replenish your skin's moisture without oil or a greasy residue. These refreshingly light, oil-free, water-based, noncomedogenic moisturizers replace depleted moisture in oily and acne-prone skin.

Directions: Apply sparingly to face to lock in moisture. Reapply as needed. Use under makeup for a smoother application and appearance.

- *Collastin Oil-Free Moisturizer for the Face*

- *Nivea Oil-Free Gel Moisturizer*

- *Nivea Visage No Oil All Moisture Hydrogel*

- *Olay Oil-Free Beauty Fluid*

- *Purpose Dual Treatment Moisture Lotion, SPF 15*
- *Stallex Hydrate and Soften, Level 1:* our lightest moisturizer.

Sunscreens for Oily/Acne-prone Skin:

Sunscreen protects you from damaging sun rays that cause sunburn, wrinkles, freckling, premature aging, and of course, skin cancer. These broad-spectrum sunscreens are oil free and noncomedogenic. So go ahead and have fun in the sun—you're protected!

Directions: Apply sparingly to face, avoiding eyelids, a half hour before sun exposure. Reapply every two hours and after swimming and perspiring.

- *Bain de Soleil Oil-Free All Day Gentle Block, SPF 30*
- *Coppertone Oil Free Waterproof Sunblock Lotion, SPF 15*
- *Neutrogena Intensified Day Moisture, SPF 15*
- *Oil of Olay Daily UV Protectant, SPF 15 Lotion*
- *Physicians Formula Oil-Free Protective Moisturizing Lotion, SPF 15*
- *Stallex Solar Protection Gel, SPF 15 (for Face):* our ultra-light sunscreen gel goes a step further and protects oily and acne-prone skin from breakouts. Very lightweight and PABA free.
- *Stallex Solar Protection Pads, SPF 30*

• • •

SKIN-CARE PROGRAM FOR COMBINATION SKIN

So, your T-zone is oily, but the rest of your face, especially your cheeks, is dry, even scaly. Combination facial skin is very common and requires special treatment. Fortunately, there are many specifically formulated products to bring combination skin back into balance.

Cleansers for Combination Skin:

Put your best face forward by keeping your skin fresh, clean, and clear. These products dissolve and wash away dirt and oil from the pores to reveal your skin's clarity, while maintaining its natural moisture.

Directions: Use two times daily and as needed to cleanse and remove excess oiliness. Gently massage with fingertips for fifteen to thirty seconds. Rinse with warm (not hot or cold) water. Pat, do not rub dry.

- *Cetaphil Lotion Cleanser*
- *Lancôme Clarifiance Oil-Free Gel Cleanser*
- *Neutrogena Deep Clean Facial Cleanser*
- *Olay Moisture Balancing Foaming Face Wash*
- *Peter Thomas Roth Combination Skin Cleansing Gel*
- *Stallex Cleanse and Purify, Level 2*

Toners for Combination Skin:

By removing residual dirt, oils, cleanser, and flakes from the skin, toners effectively complete the cleansing process without overdrying. Skin is left feeling fresh, clean, and healthy.

Directions: Wash, then pat dry. Sparingly apply toner to a thin cotton pad and gently wipe affected area. As the residual oils and cells are extracted from the skin, the pad picks up a faint hue of yellow or gray. Repeat with fresh pad until there is no color change on pad.

- *Neutrogena Deep Clean Astringent*
- *Lancôme T. Controle Instant T-Zone Mattifier*
- *Olay Refreshing Toner (Low-Alcohol Formula)*
- *Stallex Tone and Clarify, Level 2:* this mild facial toner for normal, combination, oily, or acne-prone skin cleanses and tones for fresh, clean skin all day long.

Active Products for Combination Skin:

These actives are formulated specifically for facial skin, and can help to soften, smooth, clarify, and brighten. Regular use diminishes the visible signs of aging and past sun damage, and reveals a refreshed complexion. Glycolic-acid products are used for effective facial rejuvenation and improvement of texture and color, and to reduce potential acne breakouts.

Directions: Cleanse face and pat dry. Apply product sparingly. If desired, apply a moisturizer to cheeks as needed.

- *Basis All Night Face Cream:* alpha hydroxy acids and vitamins A, E, C
- *NeoStrata Oily Skin Solution for AHA 8:* 8% glycolic acid, pH 4.0
- *Neutrogena Pore Refining Mattifier:* beta hydroxy complex
- *Purpose Alpha Hydroxy Moisture Lotion*
- *RoC Retinol Actif Pur Anti-Wrinkle Treatment, Day:* retinol, vitamin A
- *Stallex Clear Control Solution*

Moisturizers for Combination Skin:

Replenish your skin's moisture without oil or a greasy residue. These refreshingly light, oil-free, water-based, noncomedogenic moisturizers replace depleted moisture in combination skin.

Directions: Apply sparingly to face to lock in moisture. Reapply as needed.

- *Alpha-Hydroxy Oil-Free Lotion*
- *Clinique Skin Calming Moisture Mask*
- *Neutrogena Healthy Skin Face Lotion*
- *Nivea Oil-Free Gel Moisturizer*
- *Olay Original Active Hydrating Beauty Fluid*
- *Stallex Hydrate and Soften, Level 1:* won't clog pores; our lightest moisturizer.

Sunscreens for Combination Skin:

No excuses! These lightweight, broad-spectrum sunscreens are oil free and non-comedogenic. They effectively protect combination skin from the damaging rays of the sun. So for those of you who don't use sunscreen because you don't have time or because you're afraid you'll break out, remember: there are no excuses not to protect yourself.

Directions: Apply sparingly and evenly to face, avoiding eyelids, a half hour before sun exposure. Reapply every two hours and after swimming or perspiring.

- *Bain de Soleil All Day Oil-Free Waterproof Sunblock, SPF 15*
- *Clinique City Block Sheer Oil-Free Daily Face Protector, SPF 15*
- *Neutrogena No-Stick Sunscreen, SPF 30*
- *Olay Complete All Day Moisture Lotion, UV Defense, SPF 15, Combination/Oily Skin*
- *Stallex Solar Protection Lotion, SPF 15 (for Face)*

• • •

SKIN-CARE PROGRAM FOR DRY SKIN

Overexposure to sun, overuse of soap, the icy blast of winter air, moistureless indoor heat, and the very dry air on planes can leave your face itching, scaling, flaking, and thirsting for moisture. Normal water balance is so vital for healthy-looking and better-feeling skin. Here are some water-rich moisturizers—both my products and over-the-counter products—that can restore your water balance, making your skin look and feel vibrant again.

Cleansers for Dry Skin:

These specialized formulas very gently wash away dirt and oil without drying skin out. Cleansed skin is left feeling soft and smooth—not dry, tight, or irritated.

Directions: Use two times daily and as needed to cleanse your dry skin. Gently massage with fingertips for fifteen to thirty seconds. Rinse with warm (not hot or cold) water. Pat, do not rub dry.

- *Aveeno Cleansing Bar for Dry Skin*
- *Liquid Neutrogena*
- *Neutrogena Extra Gentle Cleanser*
- *Nivea Visage Gentle Cleansing Cream*
- *Olay Daily Facials Lathering Cleansing Cloths, Hydrating for Normal to Dry Skin*
- *Olay Moisture-Rich Cream Cleanser*
- *Pond's Daily Cleanser Facial Cleansing Foam*
- *Stallex Cleanse and Purify, Level 1*

Toners for Dry Skin:

Freshen up! These toners keep even sensitive or dry skin revitalized and clear all day long. They are very gentle, alcohol-free skin fresheners that remove residual dirt, oils, and flakes from skin after washing. Toners complete the cleansing step without overdrying, and leave skin fresh, clean, and healthy.

Directions: Wash, then pat dry. Sparingly apply to a thin cotton pad and gently wipe affected area. As the residual dirt, cleanser, and cells are extracted from the skin, the pad picks up a faint hue of yellow or gray. Repeat with fresh pad until there is no color change on pad.

- *Lancôme Tonique Confort*
- *Neutrogena Alcohol-Free Toner*
- *Prescriptives Immediate Glow, Skin Conditioning Tonic for Normal/Drier Skin*
- *Stallex Tone and Clarify, Level 1*

Active Products for Dry Skin:

These products remove dead cells from the skin's surface, giving you a smoother, brighter, more lustrous skin texture and color.

Directions: Cleanse face and pat dry. Apply cream sparingly, distributing evenly over entire face until fully absorbed. Apply moisturizer if desired.

- *Aqua Glycolic Face Cream:* 10% glycolic compound
- *Basis All Night Face Cream:* alpha hydroxy acids and vitamins A, E, C
- *Glytone Day Cream for Dry Skin 12:* 12% glycolic acid
- *Neutrogena Healthy Skin Anti-Wrinkle Cream:* AHAs and BHAs
- *Purpose Alpha Hydroxy Moisture Lotion*
- *Stallex Herbal Glycolic Therapy 10 Creme for Face:* contains 10% glycolic acid, natural essential oils, and herbal extracts. This is one of our starter-strength glycolic products. After using as directed for one month, you may move up to a second-strength product, *Glycolic Therapy Creme 15 for Face.*

Daytime Moisturizers for Dry Skin:

Help keep that healthy glow! These enriched facial moisturizers nourish dry skin to restore your skin's natural moisture level. They help to minimize the appearance of fine lines and wrinkles and leave your complexion visibly improved. Use under makeup for an even application and smoother appearance.

Directions: Apply sparingly to facial skin to lock in moisture. Reapply as needed.

- *Clinique Moisture Surge Treatment Formula*
- *Olay Complete Plus Ultra Rich Day Cream*
- *Stallex AM Intensive Creme Therapy:* this medium-weight

botanical facial moisturizer is excellent for more mature, non-oily skin.

- *Stallex Hydrate and Soften, Level 3*

Nighttime Moisturizers for Dry Skin:

Repair tired skin while you sleep. These night-cream formulas offer vital hydration for dry and mature facial skin. The moisturizers work hard, while you rest, to restore lost moisture, improve skin's elasticity, and reduce the appearance of fine lines and wrinkles. Wake to a complexion that's visibly improved and to healthy skin that will remain soft and supple the whole day through.

Directions: Apply to facial skin to lock in moisture. Use as often as needed.

- *Nivea Visage Nighttime Renewal Creme*
- *Olay Complete Plus Ultra Rich Night Cream*
- *Peter Thomas Roth Ceramide Ultra-Rich Night Renewal*
- *Stallex AM Intensive Creme Therapy*
- *Stallex PM Intensive Creme Therapy*
- *Stallex Supra Rich Eye Creme:* reduce the look of stress and fatigue as you rejuvenate and hydrate your eyelids.

Sunscreens for Dry Skin:

Sun protection is important for dry skin because skin can become even drier after sun exposure. Remember not to use formulations for oily or acne-prone skin because they will aggravate dry skin. The following lotions protect you from damaging rays that can cause sunburn, wrinkles, uneven skin tone, freckling, premature aging, and skin cancer. Rich in nourishing moisturizers, they are recommended for dry, mature, or sensitive skin on the body and face.

Directions: Apply generously and evenly to dry skin on the face and body, a half hour before sun exposure. Reapply every two hours and after swimming or perspiring.

- *Coppertone All-Day Moisturizing Sunblock Lotion, SPF 15 or 25*
- *Eucerin Face Protective Moisture Lotion, SPF 25*
- *Neutrogena Moisture, SPF 15*
- *Vaseline Intensive Care Moisturizing Sunblock Lotion, SPF 15 or 25*
- *Stallex Solar Protection Lotion, SPF 20 (for Body)*
- *Stallex Solar Protection Cream, SPF 25 (for Face and Body)*

• • •

SKIN-CARE PROGRAM FOR MATURE SKIN

The aging process can be traumatic to your skin and your psyche, but it doesn't have to be. The time-related natural depletion of oil and water can easily be restored to give you youthful-looking skin again, if you use the right products. Remember, it's not just the passing of time that causes the skin to age. Sunlight, cigarette smoke, and air pollutants all hasten the appearance of aging, so do your part to preserve the youthfulness of your skin!

Cleansers for Mature Skin:

These cleansers for mature and even the most sensitive skin gently but effectively cleanse skin and help you maintain a clear and radiant complexion. They very gently wash away dirt and debris without further drying skin out. Cleansed skin is left feeling soft and smooth— not dry or irritated.

Directions: Use two times daily before applying actives and/or moisturizers as needed. Gently massage with fingertips for fifteen to thirty seconds. Rinse with warm (not hot or cold) water. Pat, do not rub dry.

- *Cetaphil Lotion Cleanser*
- *Neutrogena Extra Gentle Cleanser*
- *Neutrogena Healthy Skin Anti-Wrinkle Anti-Blemish Cleanser*
- *Nivea Visage Gentle Cleansing Cream*
- *Olay Daily Renewal Cleanser:* contains BHA complex
- *Pond's Daily Cleanser Facial Cleansing Foam*
- *Stallex Cleanse and Purify, Level 1*

Toners for Mature Skin:

These alcohol-free toners help to keep mature skin revitalized and fresh all day long. They remove residual dirt, oils, cleanser, and flakes from skin after washing; they complete the cleansing step without overdrying or irritating and leave skin feeling fresh, clean, and healthy.

Directions: Wash face, then pat dry. Sparingly apply toner to a thin cotton pad and gently wipe affected area. As the residual oils and cells are extracted from the skin, the pad picks up a faint hue of yellow or gray. Repeat with fresh pad until there is no color change on pad.

- *Neutrogena Alcohol-Free Toner*
- *Stallex Tone and Clarify, Level 1*

Active Products for Mature Skin:

Glycolic acid and other actives are used for general facial rejuvenation and improvement of texture and color. These revitalizing creams, formulated specifically for mature facial skin, help to soften, smooth, clarify, and brighten skin. Regular use diminishes the visible signs of aging and past sun damage and reveals a refreshed complexion that is visibly improved, brighter, and full of youthful vitality.

Directions: Cleanse face and pat dry. Apply cream sparingly.

- *Estée Lauder Diminish Anti-Wrinkle Retinol Treatment*

- *Estée Lauder Skin Refinisher with Exfoliators*

- *Olay Regenerist Daily Regenerating Serum*

- *Peter Thomas Roth AHA 12% Hydrating Ceramide Repair Gel*

- *Pond's Dramatic Results* products

- *Prescriptives Skin Renewal Cream*

- *Stallex C Complex Rescue Serum for Face:* a combination of antioxidant vitamins C and E, glycolic acid, and green tea extract for more aggressive revitalization, smoothing, and softening of facial skin and prevention of free radical skin damage.

- *Stallex Herbal Glycolic Therapy 10 Creme for Face:* contains 10% glycolic acid, natural essential oils, and herbal extracts. This is one of our starter-strength glycolic products. After using as directed for one month, you may move up to a second-strength product, *Glycolic Therapy 15 Creme for Face.*

Moisturizers for Mature Skin:

While delivering a penetrating boost of hydration to alleviate dryness, these products also help restore missing but vital oils to complete the balance of your skin while they firm, tone, and reduce the appearance of fine lines and wrinkles. They deliver vital nutrients for more youthful, healthy, and radiant skin.

Directions: Use at night and as needed.

- *Clinique Moisture Surge Treatment Formula*

- *Estée Lauder Skin Perfecting Creme Firming Nourisher*

- *Olay Complete Plus Ultra-Rich Night Firming Cream*

- *Peter Thomas Roth Hydrating Gel*

- *Prescriptives Super Flight Cream*

- *Stallex AM Intensive Creme Therapy*

- *Stallex PM Intensive Creme Therapy*

- *Stallex Microsome Concentrate:* this is our exclusive extra-rich botanical formula.

- *Stallex Supra Rich Eye Creme*

Sunscreens for Mature Skin:

Don't run from the sun! These broad-spectrum sunscreens are specially formulated for dry, mature, or sensitive skin. They protect skin from the damaging rays that can cause sunburn, wrinkles, uneven skin tone, freckling, premature aging, and of course, skin cancer. Very rich in nourishing moisturizers, these sun-protection creams are also especially recommended for fair skin.

Directions: Apply liberally to dry skin thirty minutes before sun exposure. Reapply every two hours and after swimming or perspiring.

- *Coppertone All-Day Moisturizing Sunblock Lotion, SPF 15 or 25*

- *Estée Lauder DayWear Plus Multi Protection Anti-oxidant Creme, SPF 15*

- *Olay Complete All Day Moisture Lotion, SPF 15*

- *Stallex Solar Protection Lotion, SPF 20 (for Body)*

- *Stallex Solar Protection Cream, SPF 25 (for Face and Body)*

- *Stallex Ultimate Solar Protection Cream, SPF 45 (for Face and Body)*

SKIN-CARE PROGRAM FOR NORMAL SKIN

When the oil and water content of your skin is in balance, you have normal skin (like most of us). Normal skin, however, is not perfect skin. People with this type of skin are prone to the occasional breakout, and go through times when their skin feels itchy or dry. Just because your skin is in balance doesn't mean you can forget about a skin-care regimen— on the contrary. In order to achieve the most glowing, flawless normal-skin complexion, follow this program diligently; the results will pay off, guaranteed.

Cleansers for Normal Skin:

Put your best face forward by keeping your skin fresh, clean, and looking clear. These facial cleansers for normal skin will maintain the delicate balance of oil and water that makes this skin type so clear and free of blemishes.

Directions: Use two times daily before applying actives and as needed to cleanse and remove incidental oil, makeup, and dirt. Gently massage with fingertips for fifteen to thirty seconds. Rinse with warm (not hot or cold) water. Pat, do not rub dry.

- *Cetaphil Lotion Cleanser*
- *Clinique Rinse-Off Foaming Cleanser*
- *Estée Lauder Perfectly Clean Splash Away Foaming Cleanser*
- *Neutrogena Fresh Foaming Cleanser*
- *Olay Gentle Foaming Face Wash*
- *Prescriptives All Clean Fresh Foaming Cleanser for Normal Skin*
- *Stallex Cleanse and Purify, Level 2*

Toners for Normal Skin:

Freshen up! Keep your skin revitalized and clear all day long. These very gentle skin fresheners remove residual dirt, oils, and flakes from the skin after washing. They complete the cleansing step without overdrying, and leave skin fresh, clean, and in balance.

Directions: Wash, then pat dry. Sparingly apply toner to a thin cotton pad and gently wipe affected area. As the residual oils and cells are extracted from the skin, the pad picks up a faint hue of yellow or gray. Repeat with fresh pad until there is no color change on pad.

- *Neutrogena Alcohol-Free Toner*
- *Prescriptives Immediate Glow, Skin Conditioning Tonic for Normal/Drier Skin*
- *Stallex Tone and Clarify, Level 1*

Active Products for Normal Skin:

Glycolic acid, AHA, or BHA creams are used for general facial rejuvenation, improvement, and perfection of texture and color. These creams, formulated specifically for normal facial skin, can help to soften, smooth, clarify, and brighten your skin. Regular use diminishes the visible signs of aging and past sun damage, and reveals a refreshed complexion that is visibly improved, brighter, even colored, and full of youthful vitality.

Directions: Cleanse face and pat dry. Apply cream sparingly. Apply a moisturizer if desired.

- *Neutrogena Healthy Skin* products
- *Aqua Glycolic Face Cream:* 10% glycolic compound
- *Glytone Day Cream for Dry Skin 12:* 12% glycolic acid
- *Kinerase Cream*
- *NeoStrata Face Cream Plus, AHA 15:* 15% glycolic acid
- *Stallex Glycolic Therapy 8 Creme for Face:* This is one of our starter-strength glycolic products. After one month of use, move up to *Glycolic Therapy 10 Creme for Face* or *Glycolic Therapy 15 Creme for Face.*

Moisturizers for Normal Skin:

Help keep that healthy glow! These enriched facial moisturizers nourish skin to maintain your skin's natural moisture level. While delivering a balancing boost of hydration, they firm, tone, and reduce the appearance of fine lines and wrinkles. Use under makeup for an even application and smoother appearance.

Directions: Apply product sparingly to facial skin to lock in moisture. Reapply as needed.

- *Clinique Moisture On-Call*
- *Lancôme Aqua Fusion Lotion*
- *Neutrogena Healthy Skin Anti-Wrinkle Cream*
- *Peter Thomas Roth Ceramide Night Renewal*
- *Prescriptives Fast Acting Moisturizer for Normal Skin*
- *Stallex Hydrate and Soften, Level 2*
- *Stallex Hydrate and Soften, Level 3*
- *Stallex Supra Rich Eye Creme*

Sunscreens for Normal Skin:

Sun-protection lotions defend your skin against damaging rays that can cause sunburn, wrinkles, uneven skin tone, freckling, premature aging, and skin cancer. Rich in nourishing moisturizers, these easy-spreading lotions are recommended for normal skin. So go ahead and have fun in the sun—you're protected!

Directions: Apply generously and evenly to skin on the face and body, a half hour before sun exposure. Reapply every two hours and after swimming or perspiring.

- *Clinique City Block Sheer Oil-Free Daily Face Protector, SPF 15*
- *Coppertone All-Day Moisturizing Sunblock Lotion, SPF 15 or 25*
- *Estée Lauder DayWear Plus Multi Protection Anti-Oxidant Creme, SPF 15*
- *Neutrogena Moisture, SPF 15, Sheer Tint*

- *Olay Complete All Day Moisture Lotion, UV Defense, SPF 15, Normal Skin*

- *Stallex Solar Protection Lotion, SPF 20 (for Body)*

- *Stallex Solar Protection Cream, SPF 25 (for Face and Body)*

• • •

SKIN-CARE PROGRAM FOR SENSITIVE SKIN

Are you leery about skin-care products because they can wreak havoc on your sensitive skin? Sensitive skin may have normal or abnormal oil and water content and balance, but tends to be easily irritated by common skin-care products. Specially formulated sensitive-skin products can help keep skin reactions to a minimum.

Cleansers for Sensitive Skin:

These cleansers are for even the most sensitive skin. They gently but effectively cleanse skin and help maintain a clear and radiant complexion, by very gently washing away dirt and oil—without irritation. Skin is left feeling soft and smooth—not dry or irritated.

Directions: Use two times daily and as needed to cleanse and remove excess oiliness. Gently massage with fingertips for fifteen to thirty seconds. Rinse with warm (not hot or cold) water. Pat, do not rub dry.

- *Cetaphil Lotion Cleanser*

- *Dove Sensitive Skin Beauty Bar*

- *Estée Lauder Vérité LightLotion Cleanser*

- *Neutrogena Sensitive Skin Solutions Oil-Free Foaming Cleanser*

- *Nivea Visage Gentle Cleansing Cream*

- *Olay Daily Facials Lathering Cleansing Cloths, Soothing for Sensitive Skin*

- *Prescriptives Comfort Cleanser—Gentle Lotion for Sensitive Skin*

- *Stallex Cleanse and Purify, Level 1*

Toners for Sensitive Skin:

These toners help to keep even sensitive or dry skin revitalized and fresh all day long. They remove residual dirt, oils, cleanser, and flakes from skin after washing; they complete the cleansing step without overdrying or irritating and leave skin feeling fresh, clean, and healthy.

Directions: Wash face, then pat dry. Sparingly apply toner to a thin cotton pad and gently wipe affected area. As the residual oils and cells are extracted from the skin, the pad picks up a faint hue of yellow or gray. Repeat with fresh pad until there is no color change on pad.

- *Neutrogena Alcohol-Free Toner*

- *Stallex Tone and Clarify, Level 1*

Active Products for Sensitive Skin:

Truly sensitive skin is too sensitive for the exfoliating action of the active ingredients that so effectively improve color and texture flaws in other skin types. Products used on normal, dry, or oily skin to increase cell turnover only irritate sensitive skin. That is why I cannot, in good conscience, recommend any active products for people with this skin type; you can't be all things to all people. My own line of products does not include a glycolic active for sensitive skin. If you have sensitive skin and think you really need a product to help rejuvenate your complexion, your best bet is to schedule an appointment with your dermatologist and create a plan that is tailored to your specific sensitivities.

Moisturizers for Sensitive Skin:

Replenish your sensitive skin's moisture without oil or a greasy residue. These refreshingly light, oil-free, water-based, noncomedogenic moisturizers replace depleted moisture without added fragrances or irritants. And they won't clog pores. Use under makeup for an even application and smoother appearance.

Directions: Cleanse face and pat dry, then apply sparingly to facial skin to lock in moisture. Reapply as needed.

- *Cetaphil Moisture Lotion*
- *Clinique Skin Calming Moisture Mask*
- *Estée Lauder Vérité Calming Fluid*
- *Estée Lauder Vérité Moisture Relief Creme*
- *Lubriderm Seriously Sensitive Lotion*
- *Neutrogena Moisture for Sensitive Skin*
- *Prescriptives Redness Relief Gel*
- *Stallex Hydrate and Soften, Level 1:* our lightest moisturizer
- *Stallex Hydrate and Soften, Level 2*

Sunscreens for Sensitive Skin:

Sun protection for sensitive skin is especially important because this type of skin can easily become uncomfortable, burn, and is more prone to damage from sun exposure. Remember to look for fragrance-free and oil-free versions of popular sunscreen brands.

Directions: Apply sparingly and evenly to the face and body a half hour before sun exposure. Reapply every two hours and after swimming or perspiring.

- *Eucerin Face Protective Moisture Lotion, Fragrance Free, SPF 25*
- *Neutrogena Intensified Day Moisture, SPF 15*
- *Olay Complete All Day Moisture Lotion UV Defense for Sensitive Skin*
- *Stallex Solar Protection Cream, SPF 25 (for Face and Body):* PABA free

SKIN-CARE PRODUCTS FOR OTHER CONCERNS

Skin-care Products for Eye Concerns:

Don't let your eyes reveal age or fatigue. These soothing eye creams have a unique combination of emollients and active ingredients that penetrate the skin surrounding the eyes to hydrate, firm, and tone. The appearance of lines and wrinkles is diminished and skin looks smoother and more resilient. Not for sensitive skin. Also included are some extra-gentle eye-makeup removers for those of you who hate waking up with raccoon eyes!

- *Bobbi Brown Extra Eye Balm*
- *Bobbi Brown Eye Makeup Remover*
- *Clinique Naturally Gentle Eye Makeup Remover*
- *Estée Lauder Eyzone Repair Gel*
- *MAC Pro Eye Makeup Remover*
- *Peter Thomas Roth Power K Eye Rescue, or Oxygen Eye Rescue Cream*
- *Prescriptives Super Line Preventor+ Intensive Eye Treatment*
- *Stullex Glycolic Therapy Refining Eye Creme*
- *Stallex Supra Rich Eye Creme*

Skin-care Products for Discoloration:

Facial discolorations, from light tan colors to browns, can result from sun damage, certain medications, acne blemishes, hormones, and even picking at pimples (your mother told you not to—and she was right). They can occur during pregnancy, when some women develop "the mask of pregnancy," a discoloration of the skin on the upper cheeks, forehead, and around the eyes (see page 21). If your freckles suddenly darken, or blotches and spots spring up on your face, these lightening and fading creams will help.

- *Clinique Active White Lab Solutions* products

- *Estée Lauder WhiteLight EX* products

- *Lancôme Absolue Anti-Age Spot Serum*

- *Prescriptives Skin Tone Correcting Serum*

- *Peter Thomas Roth Potent Botanical Skin Brightening Gel Complex*

- *Stallex Epi-Peel Revitalizing Pads (for Face and Body)*

- *Stallex C Complex Rescue Serum for Face*

Skin-care Products for Sunless Tanning:

After all you've learned about the damaging effects of the sun, I hope that you aren't still rushing out to the beach with baby oil and a reflector. There are ways to achieve that "in the sun" glow without exposing your precious skin to those harmful UV rays. These products will give you an even, realistic tan; just be sure to exfoliate before you apply any of these sunless tanning products.

- *Au Courant Instant Sunless Tanning Mousse*

- *Avon Sun Self-Tanning Lotion*

- *Estée Lauder Go Bronze Plus Tinted Self-Tanner*

- *Lancôme Flash Bronzer for Medium Colour* or *Deep Colour*

- *Neutrogena Sunless Tanning Spray or Lotion*

- *Peter Thomas Roth Natural Looking Self-Tanner*

- *Prescriptives Sunsheen Bronzing Gel,* or *Allover Self Tanner*

CHAPTER

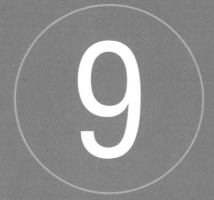

9

*"The best way to predict
your future is to create it."*

UNKNOWN

Maintain Your New Luster

CONGRATULATIONS! You have discovered how easy it is to have healthier-looking, younger-looking, better-feeling skin. Don't you wish you had known how to get the skin you always wanted sooner? Now that you know how to have beautiful skin, maintaining it will be a snap.

Continue to examine your skin monthly. As your skin quality improves, your need for products will probably change. While you'll want to continue the plan laid out in this book, you might find that you need less moisturizer or a lighter-formula active ingredient. Skin care isn't something that can be automated. Your skin is a living, changing organ. You need to monitor your progress from time to time and tweak your program occasionally.

As you go from season to season, enduring extreme temperature and humidity changes, your facial skin responds accordingly—and can have different needs. Warmer weather usually means you need lighter formulas.

Colder weather usually means drier skin, so you might need a heavier moisturizer. Hot showers and indoor heat can also contribute to dry skin during winter, and extremely cold and windy conditions might require you to use extra moisturizer every morning—whether you think you need it or not. Needless to say, when enjoying outdoor activities in any climate, remember to use sunscreen—even if the type of sunscreen you use changes, the need for it never does. Remember, snow can reflect more than 80 percent of the sun's damaging ultraviolet radiation, so look for a broad-spectrum sunscreen with an SPF of 15 or higher. Reapply it every two hours for maximum benefit. And don't forget to protect your lips: look for a lip balm with an SPF of at least 15 to prevent chapped lips.

To borrow from the United States Postal Service creed, come rain or shine, snow, sleet, or hail, sunscreen needs to be a part of your daily routine—especially if you expect to maintain your newfound luster.

I can't tell you how many times patients have come into my office after the year's first beautiful spring weekend sporting severe sunburns. The brave at heart keep their appointments with me, and the faint of heart change them for fear of the embarrassment of showing their dermatologist a severe sunburn. The reality of life is that we aren't perfect. We do get sunburns. I understand that. I never tell my patients not to go in the sun. I teach them how to protect themselves when they're in the sun. As long as you venture out your front door, you will be exposed to dangerous, harmful, ultraviolet irradiation. You already know there are elements that have caused you to have imperfect skin. Some, like genetics, you can't do much about. Others, like the sun, you have the ability to protect yourself from. Learning how is the secret to maintaining longevity in the results of your skin-care program.

There is a difference between regular and effective use of sunscreen. Regular use means applying sunscreen to your skin every day. Effective use means putting on sunscreen a half hour before you go outside, a half hour after you've been outside, and after each and every time you perspire, swim, play a set of rigorous tennis, and so on. Even if you are just sitting outside reading a book (like this one for instance), you should reapply your sunscreen

> **COLD- AND DRY-WEATHER TIPS**
>
> - *For very dry skin, try dabbing petroleum jelly on problem areas to seal in moisture.*
> - *After washing your hands, immediately apply hand cream.*
> - *Consider purchasing a cold-water humidifier to keep the humidity in your home higher during the winter.*

every two hours, because whether you know it or not, you are perspiring all the time. Perspiration you are not aware of is called insensible perspiration, which means the perspiration you are making is in balance with the evaporation of that perspiration. It comes off your skin as fast as you make it so there's no collection of the perspiration on your skin for you to notice. But your skin breathes just as your body breathes; it's called respiration, part of a very sophisticated and effective metabolic regulation of your body temperature in which you are perspiring every day, every night—all the time. And since there is no such thing as waterproof sunscreen, every time you break a sweat, you again become vulnerable to the harmful rays of the sun.

Using a higher SPF isn't the answer. All SPFs come off the skin after wear, and all sunscreens must be regularly reapplied to be effective.

Regular and effective use of sunscreen is your best defense. Sitting under an umbrella without sunscreen won't do it. Sitting in the shade without sunscreen won't do it. Sand, sidewalks, snow, and water can reflect between 75 and 80 percent of the damaging rays of the sun. The most essential step in protecting yourself or loved ones from the sun is to use sunscreen regularly and effectively.

While I have the greatest respect for the ability of sunscreens to protect the skin from both degenerative and precancerous types of sun damage, even the best intentioned and most efficient use of sunscreen will allow some sun to get through and cause a small amount of damage. Even with regular use of sunscreen, you might find that you still get a little color, a little darkening of the skin. Darkening equals damage. But the darkening of your skin that occurs with sunscreen use is much less damaging than the darkening that occurs without it. The fact that there is any change in color confirms that the sun is seeping through the sunscreen.

When the sun impacts on the skin whether the skin is unprotected or protected, whatever sun irradiation does penetrate into the skin causes the formation of dangerous chemicals called *free radicals.* Free radicals are very toxic chemicals that, through a chain of events, actually damage the DNA that causes the skin cells to be either broken or sick. Antioxidants such as vitamin C and vitamin E are chemicals that destroy free radicals. So taking these vitamins is a safety net of sorts in the fight against the sun's damaging effects. It's a second level of defense, because antioxidants can actually destroy the free radicals, which are the ultimate cause of molecular and subsequent cellular damage leading to broken or sick skin cells.

Topical vitamin C is one of the most effective and accessible antioxidants. It comes in many different topical forms. I recommend the following easy-to-find products:

- *Stallex C Complex Rescue Serum*

- *Cellex-C SkinCeuticals Vitamin C Serum*

- *Cffectives Vitamin C Serum by Obagi*

- *La Rouche Posay Active C*

- *SkinMedica Vitamin C Complex*

- *Physicians Complex C-Plus Antioxidant Serum*

- *Physician's Choice PCA pHaze15 Sérum-C*

> FACT: *When a topical vitamin C preparation starts to turn brown, it is being oxidized, so it is losing its preventative therapeutic effects.*

CHOOSE YOUR SUN CAREFULLY

Common sense tells us that the sun is strongest between the hours of 11:00 A.M. and 3:00 P.M. So if you like to run, play golf, bike ride, or participate in other outdoor activities, do so earlier or later in the day. Don't choose to be outdoors at high noon. Protect your horizontal surfaces, such as your lower lip, your shoulders, and the bridge of your nose most effectively. Women need to also pay attention to their upper chest. Any area on your body that faces upward toward the sun needs extra-special attention when it comes to sun protection. These areas are best served by wearing protective clothing—a baseball hat to protect the face or a cover-up to protect the shoulders and chest. White material that gets wet transmits most of the damaging rays of the sun, so if you are wearing a wet T-shirt, you can get sunburned right through the fabric. The color and weave of fabric plays a huge role in sun protection. High thread counts keep out more sun than low weaves; darker colored fabrics keep out more than lighter colored fabrics. But *whatever* you're wearing, always remember to wear sunscreen.

THE SMOKING GUN

Smoking is a choice that compromises what you can accomplish when it comes to restoring or preserving your skin, as discussed earlier in chapter 4. Continuing to smoke will limit how much you'll be able to maintain your new beautiful skin—besides being counterproductive to your new routine and lifestyle. If you choose to quit, you will be so much further ahead in both what you can achieve and what you can maintain. Not just with respect to color and texture issues, but also with respect to contour issues—because if you don't choose to quit, you will certainly develop smoker's lines, deep vertical lines above and below your lips, which do nothing to enhance your beauty.

In addition to the impact smoking has on color and sallowness, it diminishes the skin's ability to repair itself after any damage—especially after any damage from smoking itself. Diminished blood supply resulting from the nicotine and tars causes constriction of the blood vessels in the skin. Not smoking is as fundamental as putting on sunscreen every day—especially now that you know the dangers. It's in your control. There is simply no upside to smoking when it comes to your facial appearance.

IT CAN HAPPEN TO YOU IF YOU KNOW WHAT TO DO

To fulfill your ultimate goal of improving and maintaining your skin color, texture, and contour you have to stick to your plan—make it a part of your everyday routine. It's not complicated, and once you start seeing the results you'll want to keep them, maintain them, and even try to improve upon them. Using the five products that are right for your skin and your condition, products that work in harmony, will allow you to restore and maintain your skin's color and texture—if you use them regularly and correctly.

CHAPTER

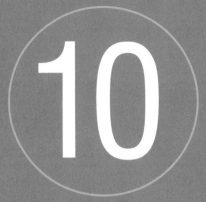

10

"What would my life be like if I had as much faith in the parts of me that were fading away as I had in the parts of me that were growing?"

DAVID WHYTE

Men's Skin Care

IN THE PAST, SKIN CARE was largely thought of as women's territory—but now the world of skin care is becoming increasingly appealing to men as well. With more men's skin-care products being produced, and our culture's desire for younger-looking skin, a new era in skin care has begun. Now more than ever, both genders are equally concerned about their appearance, and willing to take the necessary steps to maintain it.

Most men don't waste their money on unnecessary products for their skin, believing it isn't an essential part of their daily routine. It's true that men have it a little easier when it comes to taking care of their skin. For starters, men naturally exfoliate their facial skin whenever they shave, and many have shaved since they were teenagers, so they already have a head start when it comes to exfoliating and sloughing off dead cells for smoother, brighter, more even-colored skin. Men's skin care is the fastest-growing demographic in the ever-expanding world of skin care. More and more, men are beginning to understand the value of taking better care of their skin.

Most everything in this book is relevant to both men and women; however, this chapter is really dedicated to all the men out there who want to improve their facial skin. My theory behind achieving the skin you've always wanted is not gender biased, although women still dominate consumer consumption when it comes to skin care and skin-care products. If you are a man reading this book, remember that skin care is for everyone and is nothing to be ashamed of.

The truth is, I've noticed a significant increase of male patients in my own practice. Men come in to see me about cosmetic issues and procedures from fillers to lasering, hair removal, acne, and everyday skin-care issues. And, more and more, men are asking me for the same thing women have been asking for—healthier, younger-looking skin, which is mostly achieved by fixing many of the same color and texture issues women have. It's remarkable how many men are in touch with the importance of better-looking skin. But just how does men's skin differ from women's?

NOT JUST VENUS AND MARS

Often it seems that men are blessed with skin that holds on to its youth a little longer than women's skin. As men age, they embrace their wrinkles, feeling more rugged, distinguished, dashing, and elegant with a few lines around the eyes, cheeks, and forehead. While the aging process is essentially the same for both men and women—because the top layer of the skin (the epidermis) in both genders functions similarly—some differences are found in the lower layers of the skin (the dermis and the subcutaneous layer).

To begin with, skin thickness is different. Typically, in men the dermis is thicker, which explains why men's skin sometimes seems to look younger. A thicker dermis delays the development of lines and wrinkles. And conversely, in women the dermis is usually thinner, which makes women's skin look older sooner. As mentioned, men also exfoliate their skin when they shave, because the razor removes a fine layer of dead skin—every day. Hormonal balances within the skin also vary between men and women. That's why men's skin, on average, produces more oil, giving men larger pores and oilier skin. And since women's skin typically produces less oil, women tend to have smaller pores and drier skin. And *oily* skin ages more slowly.

In adolescence, men and women usually produce the same amount of sebum (the skin's natural oil), but in adulthood things change. Sebum production is higher in men than women, staying fairly constant until about the age of sixty. For women, sebum production drops sharply after menopause.

Another significant difference in men's and women's skin is their relative reactions to smoking. According to one study done in 1996, women are at greater risk of developing wrinkles from smoking than men are. Smoking shuts off the blood flow and forms stress lines, especially around the mouth. And since women's skin is usually thinner, these wrinkles show up sooner and are more apparent. I don't recollect ever seeing smoker's lines in a male patient.

One area of importance to many men is shaving. Men often ask me whether it's better to use a blade or an electric shaver. I advise them—and you—to weigh out the different factors such as facial hair and skin type, frequency of shaving, the presence of skin problems or irritations, cost, and convenience. I suggest experimenting with both methods to see which you prefer. You might find that using an electric razor leaves hair ends more ragged and split, whereas a blade razor cuts hair closer to the surface and leaves less stubble, or stubble of more uniform length, producing a smoother, closer shave. If you have skin problems such as acne, inflammation, or sensitive skin, a close shave may be less desirable since the blade can and probably will irritate and aggravate the condition, and an electric shaver will probably be preferable.

Pre-shave preparation is essential to assure a clean, close, less irritating, faster shave. Preparing for your shave includes using a cleanser that is appropriate for your skin type—a gentle cleanser for normal, dry, mature, or sensitive skin and a stronger, more effective, oil-removing cleanser for oily or combination skin. If using a blade, you'll need to choose a shaving preparation from the various types available, including gels, brushless shaving creams, aerosol foams, and brush-lathering creams. The purpose of any shaving preparation is twofold: to wet and thereby soften the beard hairs—making it easier to cut them—and to diminish the friction between the skin and razor—making shaving more comfortable. If the hairs are hard, dry, and stiff, it takes more effort and pressure to cut them, and the risk of irritation or, even worse, cutting or nicking the skin is much greater. A proper shaving preparation should soften the hairs quickly and hold them erect so that they can easily be cut.

To help reduce irritation and promote a closer, better shave, follow the steps in the shaving

Shaving Tips

THERE'S NO REASON TO HAVE IRRITATED SKIN FROM SHAVING!

Here's a shaving system that I developed for my own sensitive skin, and since then it has also helped countless grateful patients.

1. Shave in the shower, at the end of the shower, so the steam can soften your beard hairs. (Not recommended for electric razor users!)

2. Use a shaving gel rather than a foam or cream.

3. Shave *with* the grain of your hair first; then, for a closer shave, shave *against* the grain.

4. Shave only *with* the grain to avoid ingrown hairs if you are prone to them.

5. Don't shave too closely.

6. Always use a sharp blade with two or three parallel blades.

7. Consult a dermatologist if ingrown hairs resulting from shaving persist and become irritated, swollen, or painful.

tips sidebar. Shaving in the steamy environment of the shower is a great way to prevent shaving irritation. Use the appropriate cleanser for your skin type at the beginning of the shower and then rinse it off. At the end of the shower, with the water still running, use a shaving gel and shave as described, first *with* the grain, and then *against* it if you want a closer shave. In terms of shaving preparations, gels (which are my preference) and brushless shaving creams are probably superior in reducing friction and potential irritation. If you have very sensitive skin, which can be irritated by a gel, use a brushless shaving cream. Aerosol foams tend to be less viscous and less lubricating, so they may not reduce friction and irritation and provide as much slip factor in allowing your razor to effectively and painlessly do its job.

After shaving, use the same skin type–appropriate toner/astringent (which is what aftershave lotions are) that you would use for general skin care to help remove any residual debris left from the shaving products. Finally, use your skin type–appropriate moisturizer, especially in cold, dry weather.

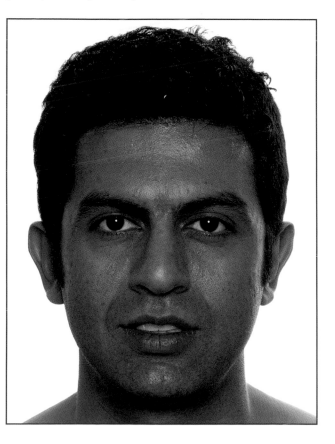

Shows glabellar texture, oily skin, and large pores.

MEN'S SKIN CARE

The good news (for men) is that, generally speaking, men have stronger skin tone than women. Thanks to male hormones, men almost never get cellulite, and they generally age better than women do. However, that does not mean that you men can ignore your skin and expect to age well. High-quality products can help a man's skin look better and age better. Aside from sunscreen—used daily—a good cleanser is a must, one that will remove all the dirt, debris, and oil that accumulates on the skin during the course of the day and overnight.

Many men skip toning the skin; however, that is a mistake. Particularly after shaving, toning can be an important step in cooling the skin and preparing the face for any moisturizer to follow.

A light but effective moisturizer will help keep the skin soft and hydrated. Add a little antioxidant power, such as vitamins A, C, and E, and you can fight free radical damage (and slow down the aging process). For razor burn or ingrown hairs, a good salicylic acid solution or a more sophisticated formulation of alpha hydroxy acids will offer dramatic results. Both acids have consistently demonstrated their ability to soften skin, improve and significantly reduce irritation from shaving, and decrease ingrown hairs.

If you have acne, any shaving procedure may be difficult and uncomfortable. Acne lesions may be nicked, resulting in bleeding or oozing. Sore, inflamed skin may be further irritated. Whiteheads may be ruptured below the skin by the razor pushing and pulling on the skin, aggravating the acne. So whether you have regular acne or experience occasional breakouts, avoid close shaves. Use an adjustable razor so that you can set it on the lightest shaving position. An electric razor is another option, since it does not shave as closely as a blade razor. If shaving irritates your skin and causes severe results, I suggest growing a beard until the acne subsides enough to allow for a clean shave.

Ingrown hairs are one of the most common complaints I hear from men regarding shaving. There are a number of factors that play a role in what causes an ingrown hair. If,

> FACT: *Men have thicker skin than women because of higher levels of testosterone. As a result, men's skin tends to sag less and produce fewer wrinkles.*

for example, you have coarse, curly hair, the closely cut ends of beard hairs may have a tendency to curve back and reenter the skin. This is a condition called *pseudofolliculitis,* which is much more common with black skin than with white skin. When the hair reenters the skin it causes an inflammatory response—just like a splinter. Shaving not only causes this condition, it aggravates it. Shaving too close or against the grain can result in clipping off whiskers beneath the skin's surface. Another factor is the roughness of the hair's surface where it has been cut; the rougher or sharper it is, the more likely the hair is to catch along the side of the follicle, or along the skin next to the follicle, and become ingrown. Using a dull blade can result in more pressure being exerted and hairs being cut on a sharp angle, making them more likely to become ingrown.

When it comes to treating breakouts, preventing wrinkles, and addressing color and texture issues or dry skin, the protocol is the same for men as it is for women (beta hydroxy acids, alpha hydroxy acids, and disinfectant for blemishes; daily sun protection with at least SPF 15 and effective UVA protection; and a good moisturizer to use when and where skin is dry).

In terms of the sun, skin is skin. UV rays are not picky. They damage men's and women's skin equally. Both men and women should embrace common sense: use sunscreen, abstain from smoking, and implement a good skin-care system. Most of us, especially you guys out there, don't use sunscreen on a consistent basis, leaving skin at risk for cancer, not to mention wrinkles. It is essential to use sunscreen to protect and preserve your skin—especially if you work outside or participate in a lot of outdoor sports activities, even coaching your kid's soccer, football, or baseball team. Any time you are exposed to the sun, you are allowing its harmful rays to penetrate your skin.

Think of your skin as having a meter that measures cumulatively any time the sun strikes the skin. Five minutes twice a day, merely going to and coming from work five days a week is almost like spending fifty minutes at the beach on the weekend. You need effective sun protection in both situations!

CHAPTER

11

"If you beat yourself up because you procrastinate, your problem is not that you procrastinate, your problem is that you beat yourself up."

VICTORIA NELSON

Botox, Collagen, and Other Fillers

YOU'VE MADE IT THROUGH THE CORE OF MY BOOK and by now you surely understand why I say "it's not just about wrinkles." However, it would have been a mistake of colossal proportion on my part not to include everything you need to know about contour defects when it comes to your facial skin. A very large portion of my professional practice is dedicated to patients who want to have smoother-looking, wrinkle-free skin—especially after their color and texture issues have been addressed and successfully eliminated. Remember, achieving the skin you've always wanted means fixing your facial problems—which are caused by a composite of color, texture, *and* contour defects.

It used to be true that cosmetic surgery and dermatological treatments were a luxury for only a few select people who could afford such "extravagances." Twenty years ago, many such treatments required long recovery periods spent in hiding and were extremely costly. These days, many of the procedures I perform daily require no downtime and can be done cost-effectively and quickly—sometimes over a lunch hour. It's common practice these days for women and men to come in for a quick superficial facial peel, a few shots of collagen, and a zap here or there for unwanted fine lines or hair. It's estimated that about 2.7 million procedures to erase facial wrinkles are performed annually, and that number will only continue to grow. As the baby boomer generation ages, they do so better than the prior generation—meaning they look better at fifty than their parents did, and therefore want to look better at sixty, seventy, and even eighty!

This chapter focuses on erasing facial contour issues including lines and wrinkles such as crow's-feet, frown lines, marionette lines, and forehead wrinkles. Most of you probably have a good understanding by this point of how the facial skin ages with time and with exposure to the sun. The net result of those two elements, plus smoking and genetics, and loss of fat and elasticity is what causes us to wrinkle and sag. Another cause of wrinkles is our natural use of our facial muscles. Our constant use of those muscles is what causes crow's-feet around the eyes (from smiling and squinting) and lines that make our faces look aged, and sometimes even stern—especially on the forehead.

Whenever I look at a skin problem, my decision as to whether or not to treat is predicated on what I call the success (benefit/risk) ratio. I weigh the upside of the procedure against the downside. First the upside: What are the relative advantages for the patient compared with the disadvantages? How much actual ultimate improvement will the patient derive, and how much of the problem actually exists on a subjective basis? Some patients see three fine lines and want their entire face lasered. To me, the benefit is outweighed by the intrinsic risk. The nature of that procedure is too severe for such a modest problem. If I laser an entire face for three lines or one hundred lines, the risk is the same, but the benefits are significantly different.

Next I weigh the downside: What is the likelihood of failure? In the spirit of the medical profession's credo "first do no harm," what are the potential side effects or adverse effects—such as scarring, discoloration, dispigmentation, or infection? What is the cost of the procedure? And finally, regarding downtime, how will the procedure influence quality of life in the postoperative period? Will the patient miss work? School? Will he/she be fully functional? How long will it take for the procedure to become indiscernible by virtue of complete healing or the ability to cover up its signs with makeup?

All of these questions are important to ask yourself before deciding on any elective cosmetic procedure. I insist that my patients do. Isn't it worth it for you to do the same?

One of my patients' chief complaints is that their skin doesn't look as good as it used to. In most cases, they immediately ask for Botox—the alleged cure-all for wrinkles. While I agree that Botox is one of the greatest advances in cosmetic dermatology, it's important to understand what Botox can and cannot accomplish. Patients who request Botox for wrinkles in appropriate facial areas will only be satisfied with the results if they have no significant color and texture problems (lucky for them). Otherwise, even though the Botox fixes their wrinkles, the patients still won't be happy with what they see in the mirror since color and texture flaws are really the cause of their dissatisfaction.

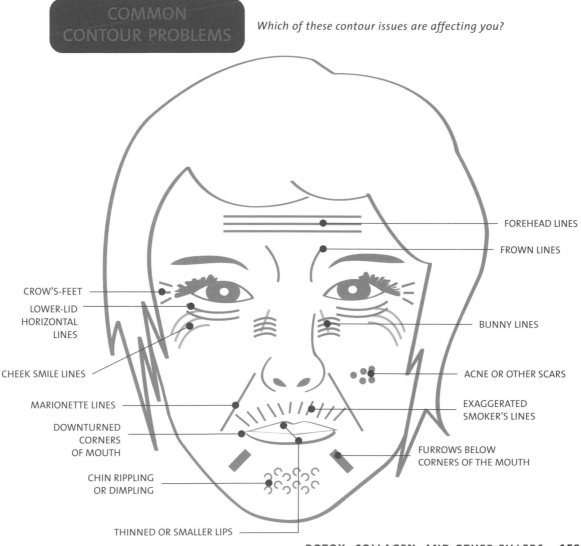

COMMON CONTOUR PROBLEMS

Which of these contour issues are affecting you?

FOREHEAD LINES

FROWN LINES

CROW'S-FEET

LOWER-LID HORIZONTAL LINES

BUNNY LINES

CHEEK SMILE LINES

ACNE OR OTHER SCARS

MARIONETTE LINES

EXAGGERATED SMOKER'S LINES

DOWNTURNED CORNERS OF MOUTH

FURROWS BELOW CORNERS OF THE MOUTH

CHIN RIPPLING OR DIMPLING

THINNED OR SMALLER LIPS

WHAT DOES BOTOX DO?

To better understand what Botox can and can't do, think of the difference between facial lines at rest (static lines) and facial lines that are visible when a muscle is being used (dynamic lines). Lines at rest are visible whether you're using a muscle or not, and while they may become more pronounced or deeper during facial expressions, they are always there. Examples are furrows or marionette lines, which come down from just above the wings of the nose to the corners of the mouth and then continue sloping diagonally toward

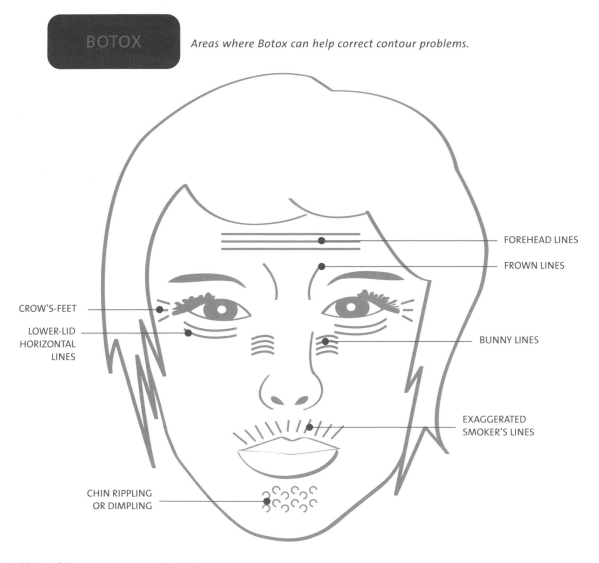

BOTOX

Areas where Botox can help correct contour problems.

FOREHEAD LINES

FROWN LINES

CROW'S-FEET

LOWER-LID HORIZONTAL LINES

BUNNY LINES

EXAGGERATED SMOKER'S LINES

CHIN RIPPLING OR DIMPLING

the center or sides of the chin. Lines on the cheeks often parallel the marionette lines, but extend in a curving fashion back toward the ear in concentric or parallel lines or arcs.

Dynamic lines are visible only when muscles are used; although they may always be there to some extent, they are deepened or worsened by muscle use. To understand why the movement of muscles causes lines in the overlying skin, think about how pulling and moving the sheet on your bed causes the overlying blanket to move. These dynamic lines are the ones Botox can help, but as you will see they are not all candidates for Botox treatment. Rule number one with Botox is you can't use it on muscles that you need, such as the cheek muscles that make you smile. While your marionette and cheek lines would improve, you wouldn't be able to smile. To me, this is not a great trade-off. On the other hand, the frown lines between your eyebrows are caused by muscles that serve no useful function, so if you want to get rid of those lines, that's a great place for Botox use.

Lines that become prominent or more prominent when making an expression can be improved by injecting Botox into the muscles controlling those lines, preventing them from become deeper and more prominent. But again, not every facial line is a candidate for Botox, and some lines may require further treatments. There may be lines on your face that are permanently etched from years of muscle contracting. You've essentially broken the elastic tissue and collagen, creating a permanent crease you simply can't get out without the use of a *filler* following the Botox treatment.

Filler material can be permanent—like silicone—or semipermanent (which I consider an oxymoron)—like Radiance (a product made up of bone material called hydroxyappatite) or Articol or Artifil (collagen in which polyethylene beads are suspended). Fillers can also be temporary, like collagen—whether bovine or human—and haluronic acid—whether from bacteria (Restylane) or from the comb of a rooster (Hylaform). These are all injected under the skin to reoccupy the volume that has been lost and the void that has been created by the loss of collagen and fat. Fillers are used for lines at rest; Botox is used for lines from *eligible* (unimportant) muscles in motion.

Despite this very simple and straightforward difference, there is a great deal of confusion surrounding the uses of fillers and Botox. Botox is a brand name of botulinum toxin, which is a protein made by the bacterium botulinum clostridium. It is made by other companies under other brand names such as Myobloc and Dysport. Myobloc is a relatively newer product and works faster than Botox, but it doesn't last as long and the results of it are more difficult to predict. Botox (and other forms of botulinum toxin) erases wrinkles because it

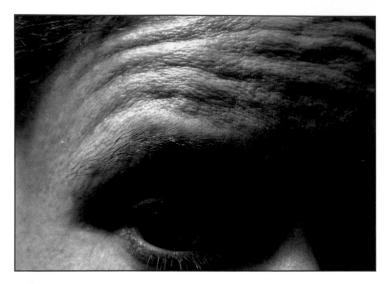

Before Botox.

temporarily prevents the release of acetylcholine, the physiologic neurotransmitter that causes muscles—including facial ones—to contract. It was first introduced by neurologists and ophthalmologists who used the toxin to treat uncontrollable eye muscles that cause the eyes to appear crossed. The doctors noticed that not only did their patients' eye-muscle spasms cease, but their facial wrinkles also softened.

Botox can get rid of the deep vertical or diagonal creases between your eyes (frown lines), eradicate crow's-feet (smile lines), and remove the deep, unpleasant horizontal forehead lines between your eyebrows and hairline. It can also erase the lines on your neck, smooth your skin texture, prevent new lines from forming, and even stop excessive sweating. This is useful to those people who perspire profusely. It's not uncommon for celebrities to have Botox injected under their arms before a big awards show so they aren't seen sweating on the red carpet. Botox can also stop excessive sweating of the palms. It is extremely effective, although using Botox for this condition can cause temporary weakening of the hand muscles because hand skin is so close to the muscles of the palms. Besides being embarrassing, hyperhidrosis, or excessive sweating, has a significant effect on quality of life. The ability to treat it is one of the most dramatic effects of Botox in terms of improving a person's daily life.

Botox is also used for various medical conditions to relax muscles and spasms. It can help prevent migraine headaches, is used for spastic paralyses in cases of stroke and cerebral palsy, and is even used for people who suffer from acid reflux by helping relax spasms of the esophageal sphincter.

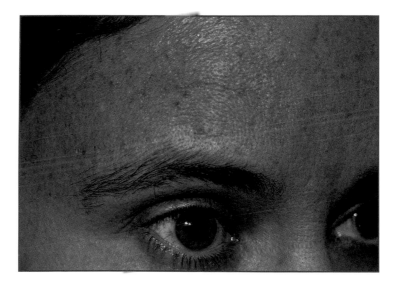

After Botox.

With Botox, specific muscles are selectively relaxed. Botox is injected with small needles into the desired muscle groups, such as the frontalis muscles, which cause the horizontal lines on the forehead; the procerous and corregator muscles, which form the line in the glabella, or frown lines between the eyes; the orbicularis oculi, which form crow's-feet; and the platysmata, which form lines in the neck. Typically, when Botox is injected to paralyze the muscle, there can be a slight burning sensation, but if done properly there should be very little (if any) bruising to the injected areas. It's important to keep your head erect and not to lie or bend down for two hours after your forehead muscles have been injected to ensure that the Botox remains in its designated site and does not migrate to the eyelid muscles—where it can cause a temporary eyelid droop. The onset of muscle paralysis takes anywhere from four to seven days, at which point 90 percent of the paralysis (and benefit) will have occurred. It may take up to two weeks for 100 percent benefit. But Botox is temporary and may wear off within three to four months, although some lucky patients maintain their improvement for up to eight or nine months. The good news and the bad news about Botox is the same: The bad news is if you like the effect, it wears off and needs to be repeated. The good news is if you don't like the Botox, it wears off and the effects go away.

Extraordinary things can be accomplished with Botox. Aside from stopping undesirable lines, Botox can prevent sagging eyebrows and dimpling and rippling in the chin area. It can raise the corners of the mouth and decrease vertical (smoker's) lines above the upper lip.

COLLAGEN AND OTHER FILLERS

Collagen makes up much of the dermis and is among the most abundant proteins in our bodies. That makes it a perfect filler material, and it is widely used to smooth certain types of wrinkles, including marionette lines and lines around the mouth, as well as to improve atrophic (pushed in) facial scars like acne and chicken pox scars. Collagen has become the most popular choice for this use. More than one million people have safely received collagen injections since the late 1970s. The most commonly used form of collagen is bovine collagen, obtained from the skin of American cows raised for this purpose. No case of animal or human disease in or from American cow collagen has ever been documented. The company that manufactures these products has a unique group of cows that has been continuously inbred since the 1970s so as to avoid introducing any new animal or protein (and hence no source of viral disease) to the herd. I can't tell you how many hooves these cows have as a result, but I can tell you they produce pure, noninfected collagen. These cows are checked on a regular basis for the presence of disease; the manufacturer has had a perfect track record of quality control for over twenty-five years.

The screening process involved in developing and producing this filler significantly limits the possibility of such an occurrence in this country; however, a few years ago when mad cow disease was a concern in Europe, bovine collagen produced and imported from Europe was banned and eliminated from use by American physicians.

Bovine collagen is available in three forms: Zyderm I, Zyderm II, and Zyplast. Zyderm I and II superficially get rid of etched-in lines and scars. Zyderm II is thicker than Zyderm I and can be used in areas where the skin is thicker. Zyplast is the most viscous or concentrated form of collagen and is injected into deeper lines, hollows, furrows, and folds. Zyderm and Zyplast are often used together in layers to effectively treat more complex contours.

To be treated with bovine collagen, you must first be tested for sensitivity or allergic reaction since it comes from a nonhuman, animal source. About 3 percent of those tested will be sensitive or allergic to bovine collagen, which can cause temporary uncomfortable red bumps and unsuitable results. Forearm skin is tested twice during a period of six weeks before treatment can be performed. The chance of developing an allergy after double testing is rare but can occur in one out of every thousand patients.

An alternative to bovine collagen is a form of human collagen made from tissue originally obtained from a human source and replicated synthetically for use. Patients who are allergic to bovine collagen or who want to avoid the six-week testing period are appropriate candidates for this type of collagen.

The human collagen I use is called Cosmoderm (for thin, superficial lines) or Cosmoplast (for deeper furrows, lines, hollows, and folds) and is produced by the same company that makes American bovine collagen. This human-derived collagen is made by a process in which there is no potential for human infectious contaminants. Collagen derived from human tissue is safe and effective and requires no allergy or sensitivity testing since it comes from a human source, so treatment can be performed immediately. Those with

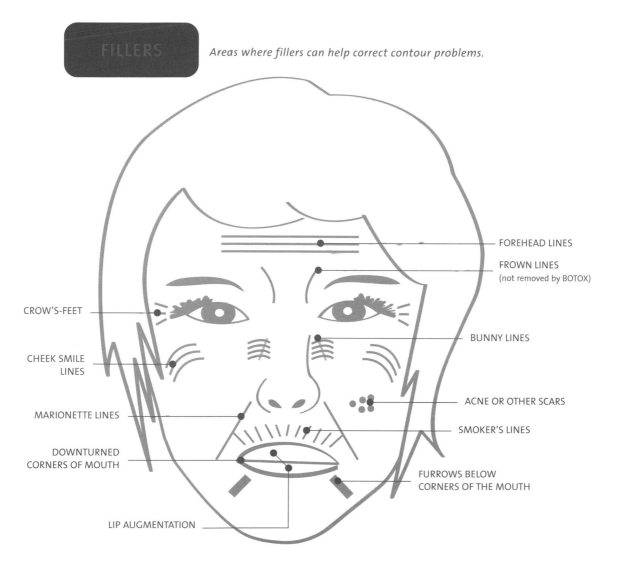

FILLERS

Areas where fillers can help correct contour problems.

FOREHEAD LINES

FROWN LINES
(not removed by BOTOX)

CROW'S-FEET

BUNNY LINES

CHEEK SMILE LINES

ACNE OR OTHER SCARS

MARIONETTE LINES

SMOKER'S LINES

DOWNTURNED CORNERS OF MOUTH

FURROWS BELOW CORNERS OF THE MOUTH

LIP AUGMENTATION

a history of autoimmune disorders such as lupus or rheumatoid arthritis are not good candidates for either bovine or human collagen treatments.

Collagen is injected just beneath the skin, and the number of injections depends on the location and severity of the wrinkles. Not all types of wrinkles are helped by collagen, but I find it to be one of the most effective, predictable, and long-lasting fillers available. Wrinkles caused by smiling and frowning, which appear around the eyes, mouth, and nose respond very well to collagen injections, as do forehead lines, crow's-feet, vertical lines above and below the lips, marionette lines, neck lines, and acne scars. Collagen is also widely used to get those full, pouty Angelina Jolie lips everyone seems to admire and desire these days. As we age, our lips get smaller and lose their shape, so enhancing the lips gives a more youthful look and helps eliminate most vertical lines, especially for smokers. Deep furrows on the forehead or cheeks can be improved but are difficult to fully eliminate. I feel that some lines make a face look more natural, especially crow's-feet, which by themselves are often seen as meaning you are smiley, friendly, approachable, and happy. They give warmth and character to the face—and in some cases, especially for men, a few lines even add a rugged, more dignified appearance.

The collagen used most often today is injected into all levels of the dermis, which makes it more effective for treating deep wrinkles and altering facial contour and superficial fine lines. The injection sites look pink and even bruised immediately after injection but return to normal within a few hours to a few days—depending on the severity of the bruising. Most of my patients can have collagen injections and return to their normal routine the same day. Small bumps might appear at first at the site of the injections, but those too will quickly subside. It is recommended to limit vigorous exercise or exposure to the sun immediately after injection.

How long collagen lasts depends on several factors. The injected collagen is gradually absorbed by the body, which does not, unfortunately, replace it. A collagen treatment can last for up to five or six months for patients between the ages of thirty and fifty, and for up to four to six months for patients in their sixties and older. How long collagen lasts also depends on how many treatments are done and whether the patient has had other cosmetic procedures. For example, if you've had a face-lift or laser resurfacing, you may need less collagen. Collagen treatments in the lips (to create fuller, larger lips) last the least time, about two months, because the deeper the collagen is placed, the faster the body absorbs and eliminates it. The quality and duration of individual results is greatly dependent on the skill of the doctor, so make sure you find a skilled cosmetic dermatologist with expertise in filler injections.

RESTYLANE AND HYLAFORM

Two other fillers popular with dermatologists today are Restylane and Hylaform, which are both hyaluronic acid. Our bodies have much of this naturally occurring sugar polysaccharide. The natural effect of this acid is to retain water, occupy volume, and enhance elasticity in the skin, thus keeping the skin looking younger. As we age, this substance naturally decreases. Restylane and Hylaform are used to correct the same defects as collagen, specifically static lines and dynamic lines not completely eliminated by Botox.

Restylane and Hylaform have become extremely popular in America because of their successful use in countries outside the United States and because they are excellent for people who are allergic to collagen. Restylane is a hyaluronic acid that is a thick gel made synthetically from bacterial sources (like Botox). Hylaform is a hyaluronic acid made from the combs of roosters. No allergy testing is required to use either hyaluronic acid product; there is an extremely small chance of an allergic reaction since hyaluronic acid is almost exactly the same from all sources, whether human, animal, or synthetic, and is not a protein. Treatment can be performed immediately with immediate results (just like human collagen). Some doctors believe Restylane lasts longer than collagen; however,

> **DO NOT HUNT FOR BARGAINS** *when it comes to fillers. These are technique-dependent procedures that should only be administered by experienced and skilled practitioners.*

it is also more painful since there is no local anesthetic mixed in (as there is in collagen) and it is significantly more expensive. All fillers should be administered by a skilled cosmetic dermatologist.

Another popular filler used today is one's own fat. It is harvested or removed from other areas of your body, processed, and then reinjected into you. It is more effective for deeper contour defects than for superficial lines and is very safe.

The FDA approved Botox for use in the glabella (frown lines) in April 2002, although it was (and still is) used as an off-label product, meaning it is used for non-FDA-approved indications. Off-label use is not an uncommon practice in cosmetic dermatology, nor in general medicine. Silicone, for example, although used for years as a filling agent with terrific results, was never FDA approved for this use. It is useful in all areas collagen is used, and lasts much longer, but I have also witnessed some horrendous reactions from using

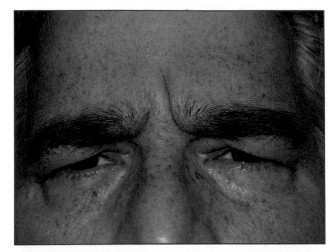

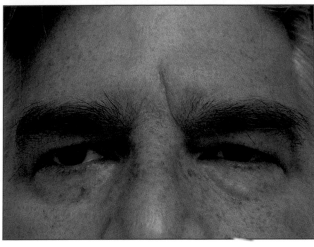

TOP: *Before treatment.*
BOTTOM: *After Botox.*
OPPOSITE PAGE: *After filler correction of residual uncorrected lines following Botox.*

silicone as filler, such as huge cysts and draining facial sores. Since silicone is a permanent filler, the sores last for years. Unfortunately, the use of impure products or the overuse of silicone, combined with bad publicity related to silicone breast implants, has really put a damper on its use as a filler over the years. That may be changing, as newer types of silicone have been introduced and are being used as effective filler.

Many products available to you these days offer false promises that they can do in a jar what Botox or fillers can do in an injection. Here's all you need to know: they can't. Wrinkles are not that receptive to creams. You can't just smear a little lotion with collagen on your face and expect results because collagen needs to be placed under the skin to have any effect. It's like trying to walk though a brick wall. You can't penetrate that wall, just as a collagen or a Botox cream can't penetrate the skin sufficiently to create a visible or worthwhile improvement in lines and wrinkles. Some products lend

FACT: *An allergic reaction to Botox is uncommon so it can be used by almost anyone, except if you're pregnant, breastfeeding, or have a neurological disease.*

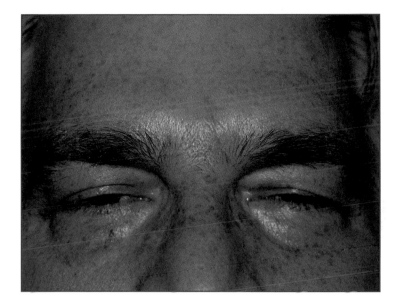

a temporary swelling effect to an area with fine lines, giving the false appearance of diminished lines. But after a few hours, those lines return. Even worse, every time you swell an area you are stretching the skin and using up the limited amount of elasticity in that area, thereby risking adding to the severity of your wrinkles as a result of overstretched skin. Remember, your wrinkles didn't form overnight, so they certainly aren't going to disappear that way—not without a shot or two in the face.

Botox is very safe when administered by a competent professional in a medical setting. Botox injections are the fastest-growing cosmetic procedure in the industry, according to the American Society for Aesthetic Plastic Surgery. In 2001 more than 1.6 million people received injections, an increase of 46 percent over the previous year. Since its FDA approval in 2002, the percentages keep rising. The benefits are terrific, with little risk involved.

CHAPTER

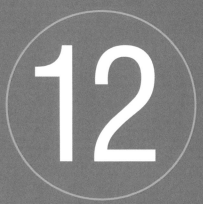

12

"All our progress is an unfolding.
You have first an instinct, then an opinion,
then a knowledge. Trust the instinct to the end."

RALPH WALDO EMERSON

Neck, Hands, and Décolletage

WHEN JUDGING AGE AND GENERAL APPEARANCE, we look not only at the face, but also at the neck, hands, and for women, the upper chest area, or décolletage. To the extent that we want to look better for a myriad of reasons, not the least of which is to feel better, there's more to improving appearance than focusing solely on the face. Women in particular find that after they have finessed the appearance of their face, their hands are still a dead giveaway of their true age. They are embarrassed by the brown splotches that connote the age of their grandmothers. When you start to see yourself from that perspective, it can be very disturbing—but it doesn't have to be, since you can take measures to prevent this from occurring and to improve already damaged skin in these areas.

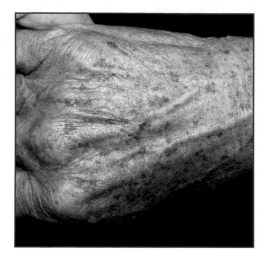

Multiple sun freckles on the back of a hand. It's a dead giveaway of age.

Your neck, the back of your hands, your forearms, and your décolletage are all areas that tell a story of time, sun, genetics, and all those factors that determine the ultimate damage to your skin. But they tell it in a less forgiving way than the face does. The skin in those areas, once it becomes damaged, doesn't have the same reparative powers the facial skin does, and it doesn't start off with the same potential to withstand and repair damage.

Your facial skin has two very unique features that enable it to withstand much more physical insult and damage than any other area of the body. It has a higher concentration of oil glands and much more elastic tissue—but by now you knew that, right? The cells of the oil glands are what we refer to as pluripotential cells, which means those cells, when stimulated to grow and divide, can become almost any other cell of the epidermis. So they are a source of new cells when old cells have been damaged or even removed. When you get a cut or a scrape, one reason your face heals so well is that there's such a high concentration of oil glands supplying these cells—so you're much less apt to get scars or even discolorations on your face than on other parts of your body.

As for those other areas, not only do they lack the elastic tissue and oil glands that the face has, they also have intrinsically thinner skin. These areas, the neck, hands, upper chest, and especially the forearms from the elbow down (which seem to get much more sun than the upper arms between the shoulder and elbow), are extremely vulnerable to sun damage. I refer to some of these areas as horizontal surfaces; the hands and the forearms are often in a horizontal or angulated position. Even the chest tends to be angled out so that the sun doesn't really glance off it. The chest certainly gets the direct impact of the sun when you lie down, while the neck has the overhang of the chin and face to shadow it a bit. That's why you don't see as many brown spots on the neck as you see on the hands or décolletage.

Skin on the neck tends to be fairly sensitive and easily irritated, whereas skin on the upper chest, hands, and forearms is more resistant to irritation—which is fortunate since

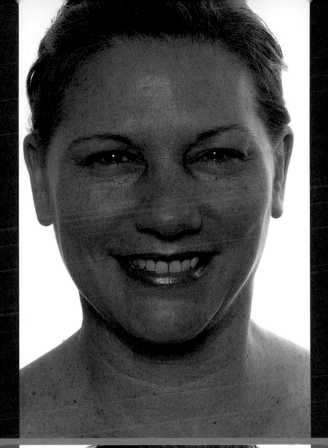

BEFORE: Most striking is the redness of the neck and décolletage (in addition to the face) accentuated by browns in the same three areas. Large pores are observed in the usual places—the middle cheeks, the cheeks next to the nose, and the area between the eyebrows. This is a good example of a Fitzpatrick type I skin type.

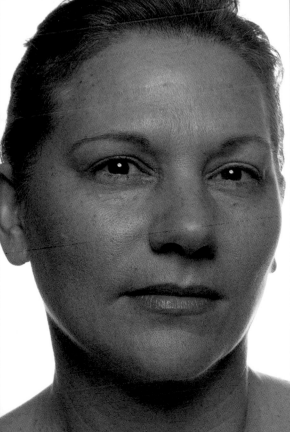

AFTER: The redness in all areas has been brought under control; the acne lesions are no longer present; and the pore sizes are significantly normalized.

the lesions there tend to be more extensive. If the face is the area most patients come to see me about, without any question the back of the hands is a close second. It's an area that takes a lot of abuse from the environment and the sun.

Both degenerative sun damage and abnormal, precancerous sun damage occur in all of these areas, so it is extremely important to pay attention to them in terms of protection and early prevention from sun damage. Start to treat these areas before you see freckles and rough and/or scaly skin. Implement an early proactive regimen preventing damage and promoting repair of what I refer to as subclinical damage. Even though you can't yet see the damage, it is there—years before it becomes visible. I always tell my patients to start treating these areas as if the damage were already there. This practice keeps the skin looking fresh and young by giving it the benefits of the medicines or topical preparations that prevent the formation of freckles on your face.

> ### ONE PECULIAR FEATURE
>
> in avid golfers is that the back of one hand often looks different from that of the other. Golfers get most of their sun exposure on the golf course while wearing a glove on one hand, so it's easy to pick them out by the number of sun freckles on the back of one hand versus that of the other.

The hormonally induced brown discolorations you get on the face from female hormones do not tend to occur on the neck, hands, or décolletage. Most of the browns you get in these areas tend to be actual sun freckles, liver spots, and age spots, which are sharply demarcated spots—as opposed to the diffuse blotches that occur on the face. Freckles in these areas tend to be larger, because there is less protection. They can be an inch or larger, rather than a quarter or an eighth of an inch, which is common for the face. The larger freckles appear most often on the chest and the back of the hands after decades of sun worship.

Red discolorations often occur on the chest, as a result of the skin having more blood vessels and being more susceptible to the breakage of those blood vessels. It's not unusual to see broken capillaries on the chest.

The sides of the neck, which are more subject to sun exposure than the front of the neck (which is shielded by the shadowing of the head) can suffer from a condition called Poikiloderma of Civatte—the appearance of stippled red and white spots caused by broken capillaries and loss of elastic tissue. People with Fitzpatrick skin types I and II are most susceptible to this condition, especially those who spend most of their time outdoors, like park rangers, construction workers, utility workers, farmers, and gardeners. This condition cannot be treated topically, but is easily treated in a dermatologist's office with lasers.

Treat the neck, hands, and décolletage exactly the same way you treat your facial skin. Follow the same four steps, skipping toner—there aren't as many oil glands in these areas so there isn't as much oil on the skin.

Wash the area with your cleanser, removing entrapped dirt and impurities, then use your active ingredient. The chest and hand skin is pretty tough and can take a higher concentration of the active ingredient without becoming irritated. The same glycolic acid you use for your facial skin will work for these areas, although you can start with a slightly higher concentration (10 percent instead of 8 percent) on the chest and hands. I recommend starting with a lower concentration on your neck since the skin there is more sensitive, or, alternatively, using the same concentration on your neck as you do on your face, but on an every-other-day basis. People with very sensitive skin may need to use an even lower strength concentration, such as those found in eye creams, just to get their skin acclimated to the regimen and to be certain their skin will not become irritated from the glycolic acid.

Choose your moisturizer according to personal preference—here, moisturizer is not necessarily predicated on your facial skin types—again, because of the paucity of oil glands. Moisturizer is a requisite for the routine, but it does not have to be the same moisturizer you use on your face.

Obviously, the need for sunscreen is the same for all three areas as it is for your face. Prevention, prevention, prevention: the three most important words in skin care. You may choose to use the same sunscreen that you use for your face, or a sunscreen that, when applied, feels less thick, like a lotion—which spreads more evenly than a cream. While my patients who use an SPF 30 make me the happiest dermatologist on Park Avenue, it's more important to me that they use sunscreen all over the sun-vulnerable parts of the body every day, even if it's SPF 15. Anything between 15 and 30 serves the purpose. As SPFs go up, the viscosity of the product often goes up, and once you get past an SPF of 30, sunscreens may begin to feel heavy and gooey, and this might become an aesthetic consideration for your skin. If the feel of a lower SPF motivates you to use it daily, I say go for it!

So remember, when it comes to taking care of the sensitive non-face regions, start early and be most aggressive on the hands and chest.

CHAPTER

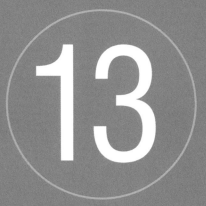

13

*"If we want peace, we must give up
the idea of conflict once and for all."*

DR. ROBERT ANTHONY

Other Procedures

WHEN IT COMES TO OUR FACIAL SKIN, we all want younger-looking, healthier skin. Addressing color and texture flaws in particular has been the focus of this book. The disappearance of lines and wrinkles is another element making up the whole picture. But there are numerous other procedures that are available to you to bring out your total radiance. All of the procedures described in this chapter are reliant on the skill of an expert physician—whether a cosmetic dermatologist, a skilled practioner, or even a qualified plastic surgeon. Flawless, beautiful skin can be yours—especially after implementing the techniques already explained to you in this book. But for those of you who want to go one step further—and who have the financial means to support that journey—I've outlined some of the more popular procedures we do in my office each and every day. Remember, none of these procedures is necessary to having the skin you've always wanted. You already know how to achieve that goal with my easy four-step program. But as effective as my program is, it does have its limitations. Many of these procedures can take your facial contour issues to the next level.

There have been incredible improvements in technology over the last decade relating to relatively noninvasive skin treatments. I have an armamentarium of technology consisting of lasers; new chemicals for injection; fillers to fill out lines; and sclerosants, which are used for sclerotherapy, the technique of destroying spider veins and varicose veins via injection. Today, many scars can be fixed by lasers (as well as by the traditional technique of cutting them out). The following pages highlight some of the more common procedures available today for addressing issues beyond color and texture problems.

FILLER MATERIAL

Filler materials are chemicals that are used to improve lines and wrinkles in three different categories: First, lines that are not suitable for treatment with Botox, since Botox can only be used to paralyze muscles that serve no useful function. Second, lines or wrinkles that, after Botox works, are still present because they have literally been etched into the surface of the skin by repeated contraction of the muscle. And third, lines at rest, which are lines that exist but are not influenced or caused by the use of your facial muscles. (It goes unsaid that these lines have not responded to the treatment of your color and texture issues.)

The gold standard of filler materials, which has been in use for well over twenty years, is bovine or cow-derived collagen. This material is extracted from the skin of cows and purified into a form of injectable collagen. I call collagen "the gold standard" because, out of the FDA-approved fillers for lines and wrinkles, it's been around the longest. As a result, we have more experience with it (I've been using it for more than twenty years) than with some of the newer products coming onto the market today—which are also safe and effective. Collagen has an excellent track record in terms of safety, efficacy, and quality control.

You've already learned that collagen resides in the dermis, or the second layer of the skin; in the cow it is the same layer of skin from which collagen is extracted. It is then purified, manufactured, and put into a syringe, at which point it can be injected into a wrinkle or scar with a very fine needle by a qualified dermatologist. A tiny amount is injected into the dermis, from which the collagen has dissipated as a result of ultraviolet damage or simply usage and breakage, thereby creating a void. The injection of the collagen reoccupies or restores the lost volume that resulted in the line or wrinkle.

Collagen comes in three different viscosities: fine (Zyderm I), medium (Zyderm II), and thick (Zyplast). There are different depths and widths to lines and wrinkles. So for a deeper contour problem, like a trough or a furrow, a deeper injection, with a thicker, more viscous material, is called for. And for very fine lines like those next to the eyes, called crow's-feet, the thinnest material in the smallest amounts is used.

The injection of collagen to improve lines and wrinkles is a technique-dependent procedure. It is strictly the skill of the physician injecting the material that determines the outcome of the procedure. If the collagen is not injected at the right level of the skin, if it's not injected in the right quantities, or not spaced properly, the results can be, at best, unsatisfactory, failing to improve the line or wrinkle (which most commonly occurs if the collagen is injected too deeply). At worst, if the collagen is injected too superficially, and in too large an amount, it can result in lumps and bumps.

There are risks involved in using bovine collagen; humans can be allergic to it. For that reason, the manufacturer recommends a skin test during which a little bit of the collagen is injected into the skin of the forearm, near the crease in front of the elbow. The area is then observed for a period of four weeks for any allergic reaction—which would result in a large, tender, red bump.

The good news and the bad news about collagen is the same. The bad news is that if you like what it's done, you have to redo it in three to six months when it wears off, or when the body literally eliminates it. And the good news is if you don't like what it's done—such as creating a bump—within three to six months that bump will disappear as the collagen is eliminated.

Four years ago, the same company that makes bovine collagen started making a human form of collagen under the names Cosmoderm (thinner, lower viscosity) and Cosmoplast (thicker, higher viscosity). The human-derived collagen has many of the same flow characteristics as bovine-derived collagen, meaning it injects and causes filling just like the bovine collagen.

Although the techniques of injection are almost identical, the advantage of human collagen is that it does not require a skin test. Since the collagen comes from our own species, allergic reactions, in theory, should not occur. Having said that, in the past two years I have had three patients who *did* appear to have brief, unimportant allergic reactions to Cosmoplast or Cosmoderm, one of whom had a redness and swelling in the injected area after about a week or two. Such a reaction is not uncommon in allergic reactions to bovine collagen. Those patients chose to be treated with different filler material thereafter.

Another important filler that has emerged is a material called hyaluronic acid, which is one of the sugars in the dermis—unlike collagen, which is a protein. Think of the structural support of the dermis as a brick wall: collagen composes the bricks and hyaluronic acid the mortar between the bricks. Hyaluronic acid is a semiliquid matrix in which the collagen is suspended, holding the collagen in place so that it can best perform its structural role— providing support for the skin.

Torn Earlobes

Women often find that as they age, they develop poor, beaten-up earlobes, which can be either partially torn or completely torn by earrings for pierced ears. If the earlobe is partially torn, the earring will not sit properly in the ear or will appear to droop down. If the lobe is completely torn, besides being unattractive, it will be impossible to wear an earring. Both of these conditions are very easily repaired by literally, in the partially torn earlobe, cutting out the hole. The lining of the piercing is skin—normal skin like you have on the outside of your body. For skin to adhere to skin, raw, exposed dermis must be opposed to raw, exposed dermis. Skin will then literally glue together by its own repair process, in which new collagen and a semiliquid matrix material form in the dermis to permanently hold the two sides of the wound together.

When performing this procedure, I literally have to cut out the lining of the hole and then sew up the resulting hole. But it has to be done in a fashion that preserves the shape of the earlobe. The type of closure I do is a plastic surgical closure, and I get terrific results.

Just as some people are tall and muscular and some people are short and skinny, some people have fat earlobes, some people have normal earlobes, and some people have very thin earlobes. The thinner the earlobe, the less material there is to work with and therefore the less able that earlobe is to support any weight, particularly the weight of an earring. So people with thinner earlobes should not wear heavy earrings. They should not wear dangling earrings, since dangling earrings invariably droop and get caught on hair, sweaters, or shirts, causing a pull on the lobe. Each time that happens, the lobe tears a little bit more until the hole is enlarged to the point that it won't provide the support needed for the cosmetic use of an earring. Also, thinner earlobes are more difficult to repair, because, again, there's just not as much material there to work with in performing the repair.

The procedure is done with local anesthesia that is no different from the local anesthesia that we use to remove growths on the skin. You'll feel a little bit of burning for a second or two, and after that, it's completely painless. The defect that we create in either cutting out the hole or—if it's torn all the way through—in removing the skin of the wedge-shaped opening is closed with stitches that stay in for seven or eight days. Suture removal is never painful. A tape bandage is worn for another week or two.

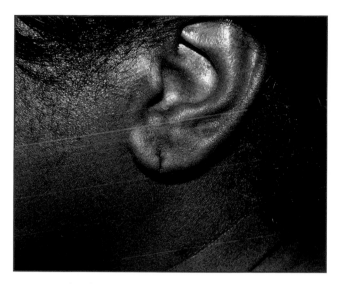

An incompletely torn earlobe can easily be repaired.

I discourage re-piercing for a period of four to six months to give the lobe the chance to completely heal and remodel. When I do re-pierce, I never re-pierce in the scar or the repair line, since scars are not nearly as strong as healthy tissue.

No two earlobes are the same. When people look at you, they can't see both earlobes at the same time anyway, so in the process of re-piercing, just as in the original process of piercing, the best piercing site is the spot that looks proper for that earlobe.

SCLEROTHERAPY

Sclerotherapy is a procedure in which chemicals are injected into unwanted blood vessels to make them disappear. Spider veins or broken capillaries are enlarged blood vessels that serve no useful purpose; as long as they're not useful, we can destroy them and not suffer any functional loss by their removal.

If you have a garden hose, and you run glue through it and step on it, you will glue the sides together, making it so water can no longer flow through the hose. That's a good way to think about sclerotherapy. It involves injecting the undesirable vessel with a material that will cause inflammation in the vessel lining. Next, compressing one side of the vessel against the opposing side will cause the inflamed walls to heal while still stuck together,

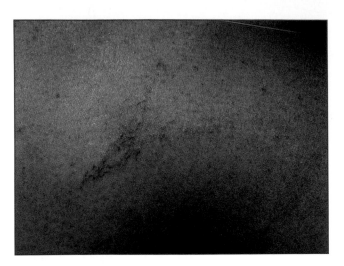

Sclerotherapy for leg spider veins.

so blood can no longer flow through the vessel. If blood can't flow through a blood vessel, the blood vessel dies and disappears as the body reabsorbs it.

The treatments are painless, despite the fact that a needle is used to inject the medicine into the vessel. Often, patients don't even realize when the injections are being performed; because the injections are so superficial, they do not stimulate pain nerves. Tight compression stockings should be worn for three days after the procedure, to obtain optimal improvement. The best stockings are panty-hose style, but they're tight and confining, so it's best to avoid this procedure in July and August, when it's very hot and humid. Immediately after the treatments, patients can resume full activities.

LASER THERAPY

Lasers are devices that emit uniquely focused light consisting of a single wavelength of energy. Daylight, or visible light, consists of a spectrum, or an array of colors of light from blue to red, which is most apparent when we see a rainbow, light going through a prism, or an angular piece of glass. Each color has a unique wavelength of energy.

Laser energy, which is used to destroy blood vessels, passes harmlessly through the epidermis and the upper layers of dermis, until it encounters blood. The blood in the blood vessel is the target for the laser energy. When the laser energy hits the blood in the blood vessel, it causes destruction of that blood, which destroys the blood vessel without damaging anything around it.

Laser Hair Removal

Different lasers are used for different targets. When I use lasers to destroy hair, I am either using lasers that target the blood vessels that supply the hair follicle or lasers that destroy the pigment in the body of the hair bulb or hair follicle, which also destroys the adjoining critical organ in the hair follicle. By destroying the critical organ, I effectively destroy the whole hair follicle. When the technique is done properly, there's no collateral damage. Nothing around the target is hurt.

The most common areas from which women have hair removed are the chin and the upper lip. The next most common area is the bikini area; next, under the arms. Beyond that, entire legs are very commonly treated. Hair on the breast is easily treated. Some women want hair between the belly button and the pubic hair removed. Literally any area on the skin can be treated with laser therapy since hair grows all over the body. Men usually seek hair removal for the back, arms, ears, and the back of the neck.

The predicate for successful laser hair removal is that the color of the hair be darker than the color of the skin—because the laser energy will be absorbed by the darker target. There is no way of removing blond hair or white hair with a laser, because the skin is intrinsically darker than the hair. The greater the difference in color between skin and hair, that is, the darker the hair with respect to the skin, the easier it is to remove. It takes anywhere from three to six treatments, but the removal of hair by laser is permanent. Patients who previously waxed tell me that laser hair removal is less painful.

It is crucial that any hair lasering be done by properly

THE VISIBLE SPECTRUM OF LIGHT

consists of about 400 different wavelengths, from 400 to 800 nanometers. A laser emits light of a single wavelength, so it has the ability to be a very smart missile. Its energy will only be absorbed by a substance or target whose absorption matches its wavelength.

Every structure has an optimal pattern or wavelength of absorption of light. (Blood vessels, which are red, are best treated with green light.) The absorption of laser energy is what causes destruction of a target, and the specificity of a laser emission is what confines the damage to the specific target—without resulting in collateral damage to other skin structures. Lasers are hugely successful because of their unique ability to specifically target only what needs to be destroyed.

trained professional. Nonprofessionals are a formula for disaster. I've seen terrible scars on patients who were treated improperly. Make sure that you are treated by somebody who is both qualified and experienced.

The best way to find a professional is by personal recommendation or by visiting the Web sites of credentialing authorities like the American Academy of Dermatology or the American Society of Laser Medicine and Surgery. Credentialing by such an authority means that the recommended professional or the recommended office has demonstrated sufficient skill and proficiency to satisfy the high standards of that authority.

Tattoo Removal

One of the reasons I became involved in laser surgery more than ten years ago was that there was an upsurge in cosmetic tattooing in an entire population disparate from bikers and Hell's Angels. It occurred to me that what these individuals thought cute and fashionable at the time would a decade later be undesirable and regrettable to them. I predicted an increase in the desire to have cosmetic tattoos removed, and that motivated me to buy my first laser.

A tattoo might seem like a good idea in the moment, but years later it may become another undesirable mar on the skin. Most of my patients seeking tattoo removal are women in their twenties and thirties with tattoos on their hands, shoulders, backs, ankles, and anterior hips. Sometimes forever is not exactly *forever* when it comes to love. And very often in these situations, a patient's new mate wants the ex-mate's name removed before things proceed. Whatever the motivation behind the removal, tattoo removal has become one of the more popular treatments in my office.

A professional tattoo has much more pigment than an amateur (or self-inflicted) tattoo, which means there's much more of a target to destroy. It takes ten to twelve treatments to destroy a professional tattoo, and maybe four to six to destroy an amateur tattoo. These treatments are performed every other month, meaning an elaborate professional tattoo can take up to two years to destroy!

Lasers are the first modality allowing for the removal of tattoos without scarring. Prior to lasers, anybody who wanted to remove a tattoo had to have a disfiguring procedure in which the skin was either cut out or dermabraded, leaving a nasty scar. Truly, the treatment was worse than the problem.

The removal process with the laser can be painful. It depends on the person's pain threshold. Sometimes I use local anesthesia, as I would use for other skin procedures. Laser tattoo removal concentrates a massive amount of energy into the skin for a fraction of a second. As the removal process progresses and there's less pigment left, there's less of a target, so there's less of an explosion as the energy hits the target. It becomes less painful. Specific lasers treat specific colors in a tattoo, but no single laser can treat every color because laser light cannot destroy its own color (so green light lasers can't destroy green tattoos).

Consequently, the more colors there are in a tattoo, the more difficult it is to eradicate it. Black is the easiest color to remove, whereas greens and blues are very difficult to remove. The hardest and trickiest colors are flesh tones.

We've talked about cosmetic tattoos, but there's another kind of tattoo: traumatic tattoos. When I was a student in medical school, I was on my way to my first neuroanatomy exam when I accidentally stuck my palm with a lead pencil. The pigment of the lead pencil remained in my skin as a black spot. That's a traumatic tattoo and it can be (and was) easily removed by a laser.

Traumatic tattoos occur when you accidentally cause yourself injury, as I did, or when you fall and scrape your body in bicycle and motorbike accidents, or when you simply trip on something. Unanticipated collisions with the ground cause dirt and gravel to get into your skin and create a tattoo. A tattoo is really caused by a foreign material being put under the skin in a small enough particle to be engulfed by scavenger cells that attempt to get rid of garbage. But the scavenger cells sit there full of the tattoo pigment and never go away. Large particles like splinters will be engulfed by scavenger cells, which attempt to rid the body of foreign material. But tattoo pigment is so fine—as is dirt from spills and falls—that the scavenger cells just sit there and fill up with the tattoo pigment, until they are replaced by permanent cells that create the tattoo.

Brown-spot and Age-spot Removal/Freckle Removal

The same laser that removes tattoos also removes brown age spots, sunspots, and liver spots. It does it with terrific efficacy, leaving no marks. The simplicity, ease, and painlessness of the procedure can sometimes appall patients in the sense of "I can't believe I didn't do this ten years ago." Patients most commonly seek treatment for the face, the back of the hands, the chest, the back of the arms, and the legs. For about six to seven days (on the face) or twelve to fourteen days (on the back of the hands, the chest, or the legs), lasering merely turns the brown spot into a purple spot. At the end of that time period, a thin black-and-blue piece of skin falls off, leaving no brown residue underneath it.

It literally takes a second or two to eradicate a freckle. Bacitracin is applied for a few days following the procedure, but there are really no side effects. The worst that can happen is that the brown discoloration will not be completely removed the first time, requiring a second treatment—which is very rare.

Laser Therapy for Broken Capillaries Including Spider Veins and Varicose Veins

Laser therapy is excellent for removing broken capillaries or spider veins. It can be used to treat areas on the face, legs, and chest—or anywhere you need it.

Let's start with the face. Those broken capillaries are thin little curved lines that almost look like the legs of a spider, which is why they're called spider veins. They typically occur on the sides of the nose but can occur anywhere on the face, and are usually effectively removed with one treatment—not requiring any anesthesia. You do feel a mild burning sensation but only very briefly.

The laser device has a cooling tip that cools the skin to about four degrees centigrade, protecting the overlying epidermis as the targeted laser energy passes through the epidermis to the upper dermis, where the spider vein resides. No bruising results. The skin can be a little bit pink for ten or fifteen minutes, but usually fades. By the time you get to where you are going, there's no evidence of any treatment. All that's changed in your appearance is the absence of your spider veins.

Whether a doctor treats spider veins on the legs with injections, which is sclerotherapy (discussed earlier), or with lasers is really a matter of personal preference. But I can tell you, even as somebody who owns sixteen lasers and thinks that lasers are better than chicken soup, I can still get rid of the spider veins on your legs better and faster with injections than with lasers. It is less painful with injections. It heals faster. And it works faster.

Laser Therapy for Hemangiomas

The same laser that treats spider veins can treat cherry spots, or cherry hemangiomas, which are those very sharply circumscribed, almost dome-shaped or flat-topped one-sixteenth to one-thirty-second of an inch red spots that you have on your arms, chest, or back. They tend to be hereditary and they increase In number with age. The treatment turns them a little bit gray, and then over the next few days they just fade and go away.

Laser Therapy for Periocular Veins

Lasers can also be used to remove larger veins on the face. Periocular veins are two to three millimeters wide and tend to occur around the eyes. Sometimes they occur on the temples or just below the lower eyelids. They are very easily treated and removed by laser therapy. The treatment is a little bit uncomfortable, consists of a few pulses from the laser, and lasts a few seconds. There are usually no side effects. The skin becomes pink or a little swollen for an hour, but the veins disappear immediately. When patients look in the mirror right after the procedure they can't believe their eyes!

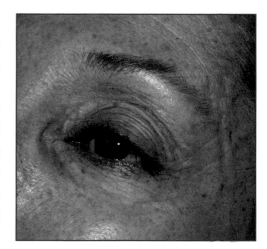

Periocular veins, which can easily be treated with laser therapy.

Laser Resurfacing

One of the earliest applications of cosmetic lasers was the removal of lines, wrinkles, and acne scars. An ablative laser literally removes the upper layers of the skin, after which healing ensues, with lines, wrinkles, and scars removed. The process of removing the upper layers of skin without burning them (that is, without using dangerous heat, which would cause scars) is called ablation; and the entire process of ablation, followed by healing—resulting in the improvement or removal of lines, wrinkles, sunspots, precancers, or scars—is called resurfacing. The carbon dioxide (CO_2) laser was the first of its kind to be adapted to ablative technology and thereby to be able to actually resurface the skin. As previously explained, lasers work by focusing a beam of amplified uniform light at a specific target in the skin. In

CO_2 laser resurfacing, the target of the laser is the water in the skin. Since the epidermis and dermis is 90 percent water, the water absorbs the laser energy, and in the process removes or ablates the upper layers of skin along with years of sunspots, wrinkles, and other remnants of accumulated damage.

The entire epidermis is removed along with the upper quarter or fifth of the dermis, depending on the condition being treated. You will leave your doctor's office literally without any outer skin (epidermis). It is the functional equivalent of a superficial or mid-second-degree burn all over your face. The skin is red and swollen (like a bad sunburn) immediately after the treatment; this is followed by the restoration of the removed skin within ten days and the fading of the red—and then pink—color within six weeks to four months after the new skin has grown in.

It became apparent to me when I started CO_2 lasering ten years ago that anything that delivered a precise amount of heat to the underportion of the skin (the dermis) without disturbing the epidermis would create some tightening of the skin. That was just intuitive and based on my empiric observations using CO_2 resurfacing over the years. This has now been proven and adapted to many nonablative lasers, which attempt to improve lines, wrinkles, and scars without ablation, or removing the overlying epidermis.

CO_2 laser resurfacing is the most dramatic laser procedure available because it nets the most dramatic results. (It's my favorite procedure to perform because my patients are more than happy with their final results and beam from ear to ear—they are truly ecstatic.)

Be forewarned, however. This procedure is not for the faint of heart—either on the part of the physician or the part of the patient, because there is a ten- to eleven-day recovery period, during which the outer skin is reformed. For the first couple of days during recovery, you're just oozing as you would ooze if you scraped your knee or suffered a second-degree burn.

Like most things in life, the bigger the benefit, the bigger the risk. The risks in using ablative lasers consist of scarring, loss of pigmentation, infections, and—under rare circumstances—long, delayed healing, which can take as much as a year and cause scarring. Fortunately, this is rare and happens in only a very small percentage of cases.

DERMABRASION

Dermabrasion is a procedure that literally abrades or grinds away all of your facial skin and embodied imperfections (scars, lines, and wrinkles) using an instrument with a very rapidly rotating wire brush. It's like a smaller version of a tool you would use to strip paint off wood. The rotating brush is moved back and forth across stretched facial skin.

The operator takes the skin down, layer by layer, until it hits bleeding levels. A skilled and experienced operator can get the layers even all over. The procedure causes the skin to bleed and then crust. Dermabrasion very effectively removes the upper layers of skin, which makes your body regenerate those layers of skin, so when you heal, the new skin is fresh and without color, texture, and (some) contour flaws. It's not the skin of a newborn baby, but it is much improved. Experienced physicians get very good results from this procedure—especially when they do a full face—but this procedure has largely been replaced by CO_2 resurfacing, which is safer and yields superior results. It can take up to two weeks before you are able to wear makeup, and several months for all of the redness to subside.

MICRODERMABRASION

Microdermabrasion involves a completely different level of depth of invasion (or *non*invasion or *micro*invasion) into the skin than does dermabrasion. It can be referred to as a Derma Peel, Power Peel, Parisian Peel, Diamond Peel, or Silk Peel—or by many other names. They are all pretty much the same procedure. Microdermabrasion is a process that is akin to a glycolic acid peel, which is a very superficial peel that only removes part of the uppermost layer of the epidermis. As the term *micro* indicates, only the uppermost layers of the accumulated, undesirable, retained cells of the epidermis are removed. The treatment helps improve skin texture; unblocks pores; removes or fades brown spots, age spots, and sunspots; and helps to reduce some fine lines.

As a microdermabrasion machine bombards the skin with thousands of sterilized aluminum-oxide crystals (the same stuff that is on sandpaper), a vacuum suction removes these particles along with the dislodged skin cells. The force at which the particles are propelled and the speed at which the device is passed over the skin determine the depth and thereby efficacy of the treatment. There's usually no bleeding, there's no penetration into the dermis, and there is no pain. Nonetheless, I recommend that only a properly trained physician, nurse, or esthetician perform this procedure.

Some Final Thoughts

YOU'VE MADE IT THROUGH THE MOST CHALLENGING part of your new journey toward beautiful skin. By now, you surely know you can look better. You know about the easy, straightforward steps you can take at home to achieve your goal of better-looking skin. I am so pleased that you have chosen to make this lifestyle change. It's so simple. Two minutes, twice a day. That's it—that's all it takes. Isn't your happiness worth four minutes a day?

If you follow the four easy steps, you will see a vast improvement in your facial skin within the first thirty days. People will wonder what's changed. They will tell you how fabulous you look. They'll ask if you got a haircut or lost some weight. In other words, they'll notice that you look *better, younger, fresher, more radiant—alive.* And when they ask what's different, you can tell them you found a virtual fountain of youth. You can explain that it was there all the time, but that now you know how to reap the benefits of taking care of your skin—because together we have bridged the gap, the disconnect between available skin-care products and your needs.

If my program works for you, I hope you'll tell a few friends—and if It doesn't, I *know* you will tell everyone. I am so confident you will love the way you look that I'm willing to stake my reputation on it.

Look, if you never practice a thing you learned from this book, you will, at the very least, walk away with the knowledge that beautiful skin is within your reach and certainly within your control. And if the only thing you do after reading this book is get that funny brown spot you've always wondered about checked out by a dermatologist, it would satisfy me to know that I have done my job in informing you on the importance of skin care.

1. How long have you been in practice?

2. Where did you attend medical school?

3. What is your specialty?

4. What hospital are you affiliated with?

5. Do you have any statistical information on the procedure I am interested in, regarding outcome, success vs. failure?

6. Have you ever had a negative result with a patient while performing the procedure I am seeking?

7. How many times have you performed the procedure I am considering?

Not too long ago, I was shopping in upstate New York when I did something I rarely do. I noticed that the manager of the store had two unusual brown spots on her upper chest. It was immediately clear to me that if she did nothing, at least one of those two spots would become a dangerous melanoma within six months. I pulled this young woman aside and explained to her that, as awkward as I felt telling her about her spots, I felt she needed to know so she could do something to prevent her dangerous precancerous moles from worsening. I encouraged her to see a dermatologist. I also told her she needed to properly research a dermatologist in her town.

When choosing a qualified dermatologist, you want to be sure they have the right credentials for the procedures you want performed. Training, reputation, and expertise are the three most important criteria to look for when selecting a dermatologist. Since so many of the procedures discussed throughout this book are reliant on a physician's skill and judgement, it's essential that the doctor you choose has both to perform your desired procedure.

Ask your friends, family, and co-workers for their recommendations. Word of mouth is the best tool a good physician has when it comes to patient care. Word of mouth works in two ways: If you love your doctor, you probably only talk about him or her when asked. But if your doctor has made an error, you likely tell anyone and everyone. Or, worst-case scenario, you don't even have to say anything to anyone—in cosmetic dermatology, the results of a physician's work say it for you.

Look for a dermatologist who is board certified by the American Board of Dermatology. Certification indicates that a dermatologist has graduated from an accredited medical school, completed at least one year of internship and another three years of residency as a dermatologist, and passed a very difficult three-day examination given by the board.

You can read about a physician's education, credentials, training, certifications, medical school, and licensure by doing a Web search on the doctor.

Once you've selected a dermatologist, don't be afraid to ask questions during your initial consultation. Share your vision and expectations with that doctor. Make sure he or she understands what you are looking for in results. You will get a good feel for how this doctor communicates with patients. Be certain you both share the same vision. If you feel uncomfortable, you have the choice to walk out of the office without having a procedure. Skin care is a sensitive topic for most people. If your doctor doesn't understand your needs or doesn't listen to you, find another doctor.

Most dermatologists provide helpful procedure brochures in waiting rooms and examination rooms. Take the time to read about procedures you are thinking about. You will get a very good description of the work you are considering and of what the process entails. It's also a great source for coming up with questions you may not have thought of in advance. Use your questions as a framework to get to know the doctor, to build trust and comfort, and to measure his or her style. The doctor is there to help you. Be direct, be intelligent, and don't worry that you are asking too many questions. I have a sign in my office that reads, "Asking dumb questions is much easier than correcting dumb mistakes." I couldn't have said it better!

I want to thank you for reading my book. It is the culmination of nearly thirty years of my life's work. I am truly lucky to practice my passion each and every day. I have friends who are cardiologists, gynecologists, and plastic surgeons. Whenever we are at a professional function, my colleagues marvel that my beeper seems to go off more frequently than any one else's. It's not that I am more popular. I believe it's because I have a very personal approach in my practice and my patients know they can call on me twenty-four/seven. You may not be one of my patients, but I hope that reading this book, in some small way, has made you feel that you, too, can depend on my advice—with the added luxury of being able to go back and read any section at any time.

One of my favorite sayings is "You are either part of the problem, or you are part of the solution." I raised my son, Stuart, on this advice; it has helped him make sound choices on his life journey. After reading this book, it is my sincerest hope that you, too, will become part of the solution. The skin you've always wanted is thirty days away. It's time to stop being part of the problem and become part of the solution—the Schultz solution. Good luck on your journey. I will be with you every step of the way.

ACKNOWLEDGMENTS

I would like to thank a number of people who have had a vital impact both on my career as a physician and in the genesis and creation of this book, which is intimately related to my career as a cosmetic dermatologist.

My late father, Sidney, who impressed upon me that in a race, as in life, you are either part of the pack or you are ahead of the pack. And so I learned the importance of not seeing other people's heels.

Stuart, my son, my best friend, my moral compass, my reason for being, my root inspiration, my pride and my love. What a great kid—and now, young adult—but more importantly, what a sensitive, caring person (after whom my skin-care line, Stallex for Perfect Skin, is named).

Gwen Schultz, who has loved, stood by, and supported me for more than thirty years, for better and for worse, and who, when it was time for me to choose a specialty, told me in her consistently supportive mantra, "Follow your heart." The rest is history. My dermatology office, described by patients and visitors as wonderfully soothing and calming, is a product of her style and taste, as are many aspects of the design and packaging of Stallex.

Alan Altman, first friend, then attorney and legal counselor, then life-issues advisor, then deal maker, then amateur but effective psychiatrist, and one of the two clearest, most incisive thinkers (the other being my coauthor) that I've ever known.

Glyn Eppy and Domenic Lopergolo of the Design Spot—they exude what can only be described as creative genius dressed in haute couture, the net result of which is just drop-dead gorgeous, exciting, innovative designs. They have designed everything that has been so well received by my patients and public in the past six years, from the Stallex packaging and labeling—which earned them the recognition and pride of being one of five finalists at the International Packaging Competition in 2003—to all of the brochures, stationary exhibits, and design elements that have gone into the incredibly beautiful presentation of everything related to Stallex and Park Avenue Skin Care.

Truitt Bell and Gus Bezas, preeminent skin-care-industry professionals, for their unconditional support and encouragement in validating the importance of this book's message and its contribution to the understanding of skin care by women and men everywhere.

Chris Helmbrecht, founder of http://www.Cygen.net, who has become such an important friend but who started and remains the Web master and designer of the Stallex and Park Avenue Skin Care Web sites, which are pivotal vehicles for disseminating information, first about skin-care issues—written in a plain, simple, easy-to-understand style—and second, about Stallex for Perfect Skin products—for patients, readers, and anyone who uses these products or wants to get on track with their skin care.

John Kulesza, for sharing with me his incredible fund of knowledge of the marriage of chemistry, pharmacology, and clinical therapeutics, which has been so enlightening and helpful to me in better treating, improving, and curing many of my patients' skin-care problems.

The Park Avenue Skin Care team, *each* of whom is indispensable. I'd like to thank Joyce Coplan—without her unrelenting help and unconditional support, this book would have been profoundly more difficult for me, as would my day-to-day existence. Her sound judgment, solicited and sometimes unsolicited advice, know-how, perseverance, and style are so important to me—not to mention her very warm smile. Thanks also to Angela Favale; Debbie Case, RN; Deborah VanCoughnett, RPA; Dianne Funes; Gina Alvarado; Marina Konstantinova; Monica O'Neill; and Stephanie Dockstader. They share a devotion and sensitivity, that makes our patients feel welcome, appreciated, and important (as they are). I am very lucky to work with such a terrific and cohesive family of caring and capable professionals.

The late Leon Hess, who had the unique ability to make anyone he spoke to feel like the most important person in the room; his approach was so inspiring and instructive in helping me to communicate with and create a comfort level with my patients.

The team at STC—especially the publisher, Leslie Stoker, and my wonderful editor, Jennifer Levesque. Thank you for taking a chance on this book and for believing in the message we all agree was important to convey. Your support and enthusiasm are so greatly appreciated.

Our research assistants, Adam Mitchell and Emily Copeland, for their tireless efforts, contagious curiosity, enthusiasm, accuracy, and youthful energy in researching and integrating countless multimedia sources.

Lastly, and most importantly, my coauthor, Laura Morton. When people do things particularly well, they make it look easy, but in fact, having been through this experience with Laura, I know that writing a book is a very difficult, complex procedure, and yet she does it with such finesse, expertise, and ability that she makes it look easy. I want to extend a heartfelt thanks to Ms. Morton for her enthusiasm, commitment, and professionalism.

For further information about Stallex for Perfect Skin skin-care products, please visit our Web site at http://stallexskincare.com.

GLOSSARY

ACID: in skin-care terms, anything with a pH 1 to a pH 7. A weak acid is less irritating to skin than a weak alkali because normal skin has an acidity level of 5.5–6.5.

ACTINIC KERATOSIS: a sharply outlined, red- or skin-colored scaly lesion (sore) associated with long-term sun exposure. These lesions typically appear on the face, neck, ears, hands, forearm, and the upper trunks of middle-aged or elderly individuals, especially those with fair complexions. They are premalignant and, if left untreated, may become a type of skin cancer known as squamous-cell carcinoma.

AGE SPOTS: (also called liver spots, sunspots, or solar lentigines) flat brown areas usually found on the face, hands, back, and feet. They are associated with aging, but chronic sun exposure is a major cause. They are easily and safely removed by a dermatologist.

ALPHA HYDROXY ACIDS (AHAS): any of various organic acids with a similar structure that are often referred to as "fruit acids" because many of these compounds are found in fruits—besides being in other foods such as milk and sugarcane. AHAs are used in skin-care products such as facial peels because of their ability to soften the skin and cause shedding of the top layers of dead skin cells. Examples of AHAs commonly found in skin-care products include glycolic acid and lactic acid.

ANGIOMA: a benign tumor in the skin, made up of blood or lymph vessels.

ANTIOXIDANT: any synthetic or natural substance that is capable of counteracting the damaging effects of oxidation (when oxygen molecules break down) in body tissues. Oxidation produces potentially harmful molecules such as free radicals.

Antioxidants convert free radicals into harmless waste products. Examples of antioxidants are vitamins A, C, E, and selenium.

ASCORBIC ACID: vitamin C, added to skincare products as an antioxidant.

ASTRINGENT: a cosmetic that helps cleanse the skin and temporarily tightens the pores. Astringents are very effective in removing oils and soap residue from the skin. This is the same as toner or freshener.

BASAL CELLS: type of cells found in the outer layer (epidermis) of skin. Basal cells are responsible for producing the overlying squamous cells in the skin.

BASAL-CELL CARCINOMA: the most common type of skin cancer, it arises from the basal cells of the epidermis (outer layer of skin). Fair-skinned individuals who don't tan well are highly susceptible to developing basal-cell carcinoma with prolonged sun exposure. It does not invade the bloodstream or move to other parts of the body, but can grow extensively on the skin surface and may, in rare cases, invade deeply, causing extensive destruction of muscle and bone. It is characterized by small shiny raised bumps on the skin that may bleed.

BETA HYDROXY ACID (BHA): salicylic acid, the only BHA, is an organic acid that is commonly used in skin-care products. It is found in facial peels because of its ability to soften the skin and cause shedding of the top layers of dead skin cells. It is also used in skin-care products to enhance the absorption and penetration into the skin of other ingredients that are in the same cosmetic formulation.

BLACKHEAD: a lesion seen in acne that is caused when the hair follicle becomes

filled with a plug of oil, bacteria, and cells but remains open to the skin surface. Because the plug is open and exposed to air, oxidation of one of the components of the plug causes the surface of the plug to turn black.

BOIL: tender red swollen areas that form around hair follicles in the skin.

BOTULINUM TOXIN TYPE A (BOTOX): a chemical derived from bacteria that, when injected into specific muscles, immobilizes those muscles. If they are facial muscles it will prevent them from forming wrinkles and furrows. This paralysis relaxes facial muscles for three to six months.

CARCINOMA: a name for any cancer that develops from cells that cover the outside and inside surfaces of the body, for example, the skin cells and cells that line the stomach and intestines.

CELLULITE: deposits of fat and fibrous tissue causing dimpling of the skin overlying a fatty area of the body.

COLLAGEN: the Greek word for "glue." Collagen is a protein that serves as the support structure for the skin and all other connective tissues. In human skin, collagen fibers comprise more than 70 percent of the dry weight of the dermis.

COMEDOGENIC: term used to describe a pore-blocking ingredient that can cause blackheads or whiteheads.

COMEDONES: enlarged hair follicles or pores filled with sebum (oil), dead cells, and bacteria. If they are open to the skin surface, they are known as blackheads, or open comedones. If they are closed to the skin surface, they are known as whiteheads, or closed comedones.

CYST: a deep lesion that is filled with pus or other contents, such as keratin and oil.

CYSTIC ACNE: a severe form of acne distinguished by large cysts and eventual scarring.

DERMATITIS: inflammation of the skin associated with a number of skin conditions.

DERMIS: the middle layer of the skin, beneath the epidermis. The dermis is largely fibrous and contains collagen and elastin, the proteins responsible for the support and elasticity of the skin. The dermis also contains blood vessels, nerves, lymph vessels, sweat glands, and hair follicles.

ECZEMA: (also called atopic dermatitis) a skin inflammation that is characterized by itching, scaling, and thickening of the skin, and is usually located on the face, elbows, knees, and arms.

ELASTIN: a connective tissue protein that forms resilient fibers in the skin and allows the skin to snap back when stretched.

EMOLLIENT: an agent that will make the skin soft and smooth by increasing hydration, or water content, of the outer layer of skin through enhancing water retention. Petrolatum is an example of an emollient that is widely used in products applied to the skin.

EMULSION: a preparation of one liquid that is distributed in small droplets throughout another liquid. For instance, water droplets may be dispersed throughout oil, or oil may be dispersed throughout water. Creams and lotions require the presence of an emulsifier to allow the combination of water and oils.

EPIDERMIS: the outer layer of skin, which covers the entire body and is only about as thick as a single sheet of paper.

EXFOLIANT: an agent that causes exfoliation, or shedding of dead skin cells. There are chemical exfoliants (alpha hydroxy acids, beta hydroxy acids, and polyhydroxy acids) and physical exfoliants (facial scrubs). The latter are lotions or creams containing small, rough particles that are rubbed vigorously over the skin to remove the top layers of cells. Microdermabrasion is also a form of physical exfoliation.

FILLER INJECTIONS: most commonly collagen (a gel-like substance derived from purified animal tissue, and fat harvested from a patient's thigh or abdomen) injected into the skin to plump up facial lines, wrinkles, acne scars, or any other depressed or sunken-in area.

FOLLICULITIS: an inflammation of the hair follicles due to an infection or irritation.

FREE RADICALS: unstable molecules in our bodies that attack other molecules, setting up reactions that are damaging to healthy cells. Free radicals are created when oxygen molecules break down due to metabolism, radiation, exercise, ozone exposure, cancer-causing substances (carcinogens), or other environmental toxins, especially ultraviolet irradiation from the sun.

GLYCOLIC ACID: the simplest and smallest of a group of naturally occurring acids that collectively are known as alpha hydroxy acids, or AHAs. Many of these acids are found in fruits and other foods. Glycolic acid itself comes from sugarcane. Used as a chemical peel for sloughing off superficial dead skin cells to reveal a fresher complexion, and to treat or prevent acne breakouts.

HYDROQUINONE: an agent that causes depigmentation (lightening) of dark spots on the skin by interfering with the production of new pigment.

HYPERPIGMENTATION: pigmentation producing darker-than-usual skin.

HYPERTROPHIC SCARRING: caused by the excessive formation of new tissue during wound healing. Hypertrophic scars are hard and raised; different than keloids, they are confined to the area of the original injury.

HYPOALLERGENIC: a term commonly seen on skin-care products to indicate the improbability of allergic reactions. Irritation or redness may still occur (these are not allergic reactions) if an individual has sensitive skin. Products are classified as hypoallergenic if fewer than five people per thousand have been shown to have allergic reactions to the product.

KELOIDS: formed when the scar from a wound or deep cut extends and spreads beyond the size of the original wound. Keloids vary in shape, size, and location, and are found most often in darkly pigmented skin. Common sites of occurrence are the earlobes, neck, forearms, and hands.

KERATIN: the name for a group of proteins made by the keratinocytes in the skin. It is the principal component of the epidermis, hair, and nails. Keratin serves as a protective barrier for the body.

KERATINOCYTES: the most abundant cells in the epidermis (95 percent), keratinocytes make the proteins known as keratin.

LASER RESURFACING: uses high-energy light to peel away sun-damaged skin, wrinkles, scars, or birthmarks. Laser resurfacing may be used to minimize wrinkles and fine scars.

LENTIGO: an age spot, sunspot, or liver spot.

LIVER SPOT: common name for a flat brown spot frequently found on the face and the backs of the hands, caused by exposure to sunlight. Rarely seen in people with darkly pigmented skin, it has no relation to the liver. Also known as an age spot or by the technical name *solar lentigo*.

MALIGNANT: a term used to reference cancer. Malignant can also refer to a disease that is resistant to therapy, very severe, and frequently fatal.

MELANIN: a brown pigment produced by pigment-producing skin cells (melanocytes). An increased amount of melanin results in a darkening of the skin, or a tan, following exposure to the ultraviolet rays of the sun.

MELANOCYTES: skin cells located in the basal layer at the epidermis that produce the pigment known as melanin, which gives color to the skin.

MELANOMA: a type of skin cancer arising from the pigment-producing skin cells (melanocytes). The tumors typically appear as irregularly shaped flat or raised growths that are dark brown, black, or tan in color and asymmetric, with irregular borders. The incidence for melanoma is increasing at an alarming rate, but it can be cured when detected early. Risk factors include a family history of melanoma, severe sunburn before age fourteen, red hair and freckling, inability to tan, numerous moles on the skin, and unusually shaped or colored moles.

MELASMA: the Greek word for "black spot." Melasma is a dyschromia that results in an area of light or dark brown hyperpigmented skin occurring in areas of the body that are exposed to sunlight, most often the face. Melasma tends to be most common in women who are pregnant or taking birth control pills, whose skin is exposed to sunlight.

MICRODERMABRASION: superficial peeling with minimal risk of dyspigmentation or scarring that is achieved by projecting aluminum microcrystals onto the skin (also known by the names Power Peel, Europeel, Parisian Peel, and Derma Peel); safe for all skin types except sensitive skin.

MOLES: small skin marks caused by pigment-producing cells in the skin.

NEVUS: a mole; a pigmented lesion that may be smooth or rough, raised or flat, regularly shaped or irregularly shaped, colored or noncolored.

NODULE: (also called papule) a solid raised bump greater than one centimeter.

NONCOMEDOGENIC: a term commonly seen on skin-care products that indicates the product was tested and does not cause the pores of the skin to become plugged and form comedones (blackheads and whiteheads), as seen in acne.

PAPULE: the Latin word for "pimple." It is a small, solid, raised lesion on the skin.

PHOTOAGING: the damage that accumulates in the skin from years of excessive and chronic sun exposure. Photoaging accounts for much of the "old look" associated with aging.

PHOTODAMAGE: the cumulative effects of sun exposure. The severity depends on the duration and intensity of sun exposure and on the skin type of the individual. It appears as blotchiness, uneven tones, rough texture, wrinkles, fine lines, and broken capillaries.

PHOTOSENSITIVITY: an abnormal sensitivity to sunlight, usually due to the action of certain drugs. When a label states that a drug may cause photosensitivity, an individual may get a sunburn in a much shorter period of time than is typical for that individual.

PIGMENT: any substance whose presence in the tissues or cells of animals or plants colors them. Melanin is the pigment produced by skin cells (melanocytes) that colors the skin.

PITYRIASIS ROSEA: a common skin condition characterized by scaly, pink, inflamed skin.

PORT-WINE STAINS: (also called nevi flammeus) permanent, flat, pink, red, or purple marks on the skin.

PUSTULE: a pimplelike swelling of the skin that contains pus.

RETINOIC ACID: vitamin A acid, also known as tretinoin, commonly used in the treatment of acne and photodamage. It improves fine and coarse wrinkling, may lighten age spots, helps the skin feel smoother, and increases production of collagen and elastic fibers.

RETINOL: a derivative of vitamin A that is used in skin-care products. It is weaker than retinoic acid but penetrates the skin well and is less irritating.

ROSACEA: a chronic, inflammatory, acnelike disease of the skin, usually involving the middle third of the face. Rosacea is characterized by persistent redness (flushing and blushing) and often by small visible blood vessels (telangiectasias), with episodes of papules and pustules.

SALICYLIC ACID: a keratolytic drug (a drug that removes the outer layer of skin) that is used to treat various skin conditions.

SCALES: dead skin cells that look like flakes or dry skin.

SCLEROTHERAPY: a process whereby a concentrated solution of salt water or other substance (salerusant) is injected into a vein. This induces inflammation and eventually causes the vessel to collapse and close. The vein becomes invisible, since it no longer carries blood. Sclerotherapy is used as a cosmetic treatment for spider veins.

SEBACEOUS GLANDS: glands in the dermis of the skin that usually open into the hair follicles and release sebum.

SEBORRHEA: overactivity of the sebaceous glands that results in an excessive amount of sebum. This results in the appearance of greasy or oily skin (especially on the face) and hair.

SEBORRHEIC DERMATITIS: a chronic inflammatory disease of the skin characterized by redness, itching, and scaling, occurring in regions where the sebaceous glands are most active, such as the face, body folds, and especially the scalp, where there is shedding of the scales (dandruff).

SEBORRHEIC KERATOSIS: flesh-colored, greasy-looking, yellow, brown, or black wartlike papules.

SKIN CANCER: see basal-cell carcinoma, melanoma, and squamous-cell carcinoma.

SKIN RESURFACING: removal of the outer layer of the skin using abrasion, chemicals, or a laser, resulting in smoother and less wrinkled skin.

SKIN TAGS: soft, small, flesh-colored skin flaps on the neck, armpits, or groin.

SPF: sun protection factor. Manufacturers of sunscreen products that protect against ultraviolet B (UVB) radiation are required to label their products with an SPF value, which can range from 4 to 60 (some may be higher). The higher the number, the better the product is for protection against ultraviolet UVB radiation. The term *SPF* is not used to describe sunscreens that protect against UVA radiation.

SPIDER ANGIOMA: a bright red blanchable papule with red blanchable tentacles radiating from it.

SPIDER VEINS: tiny broken dilated blood vessels on the face and other body parts, usually caused by the sun's radiation or by female hormones.

SQUAMOUS CELLS: (also called keratinocytes) the primary cell types found in the epidermis, the outer layer of skin.

SQUAMOUS-CELL CARCINOMA: a skin cancer that is characterized by red, scaly skin that becomes an open sore. It arises from the skin cells known as the keratinocytes, the most common cells of the epidermis. It may resemble basal-cell carcinoma but is less common—affecting about 15–20 percent of patients with skin cancer—and tends to enlarge more rapidly. Fair-skinned individuals who don't tan well are highly susceptible to developing squamous-cell carcinoma with prolonged sun exposure.

SUBCUTIS: the deepest (third) layer of skin; also known as the subcutaneous layer.

SURFACTANTS: compounds that break up oil, grease, and water into small particles so they cleanse better. They can be synthetic or natural (such as from coconut oil). Some are very harsh on the skin.

TONER: see astringent.

TRETINOIN: a vitamin A acid, also known as all-trans retinoic acid, commonly used in the treatment of acne and photodamage.

TUMOR: a mass or lump that can be felt with the hand or seen with the naked eye. Not all tumors are cancers, and not all cancers are tumors.

UVA: ultraviolet radiation with the longest wavelengths—320 to 400 nanometers. Long-wave UVA radiation penetrates the skin more deeply and causes less burning, but is believed to be responsible for premature aging and wrinkling. UVA is called the "tanning" spectrum of ultraviolet radiation and is the radiation emitted by tanning beds.

UVB: ultraviolet radiation with wavelengths between 290 and 320 nanometers. Much of the UVB radiation is absorbed by the ozone layer and never reaches the earth. UVB is referred to as the "sunburn" spectrum of ultraviolet radiation since the rays cause reddening of the skin and do not penetrate to the deeper layers of the skin.

UVC: ultraviolet radiation with the shortest wavelengths—200 to 290 nanometers. These rays are completely absorbed by the ozone and are not present in natural sunlight.

VARICOSE VEINS: permanent enlargement and twisting of veins, most commonly seen in the legs. The veins appear large and swollen as a result of a problem with the valves in the veins. There is a hereditary influence in some individuals, and a predisposition among people in jobs that require long periods of standing. They also tend to occur during pregnancy.

VITILIGO: a skin disorder characterized by smooth white patches on various parts of the body caused by the loss of the natural pigment. The pigment-producing cells are completely lost in the white patches due to an autoimmune process.

WHITEHEAD: a lesion seen in acne that is caused when the hair follicle becomes filled with a plug of oil, bacteria, and cells and remains closed to the skin surface.

SELECTED SOURCES

"Add More Sunscreen, Eat Less Fat." *Diabetes Forecast* 29, no. 7 (July 1996):17(1).

American Academy of Dermatology, Public Resources. "Actinic Keratoses and Skin Cancer: How Are They Different?" 2003. http://www.aad.org/July04_aks.html (15 July 2004).

American Academy of Dermatology, *AgingSkinNet Glossary*. 2002. http://www.skincarephysicians.com/agingskinnet/Glossary.html (4 August 2004).

American Academy of Dermatology, Public Resources. "Black Skin." 1987. http://www.aad.org/pamphlets/black.html (15 July 2004).

American Academy of Dermatology, Public Resources. "Combination Therapies Offer New Management Options for Acne and Rosacea." 2001. http://www.aad.org/PressReleases/combination.html (15 July 2004).

American Academy of Dermatology, Public Resources. "Fact Sheet: Actinic Keratoses and Skin Cancer." 2003. http://www.aad.org/SkinCancerNews/FactSheet_AK.html (15 July 2004).

American Academy of Dermatology, Find a Dermatologist. "Dermatologist Profile: Neal B. Schultz, MD." 2004. http://www.aad.org/ ZDermSP/DermSearch/profile.php?prof_id=553 (27 July 2004).

American Academy of Dermatology, Public Resources. "Frequently Asked Questions about Actinic Keratoses and Skin Cancer." 2003. http://www.aad.org/SkinCancerNews/FAQ_AK_SC.html (15 July 2004).

American Academy of Dermatology. "Separating the Myth from the Fact about Dry Winter Skin." December 4, 2002. http://www.aad.org (4 Nov 2004).

American Academy of Dermatology, Public Resources. "Dermatologists Dis-'Patch' Dark Side of Melasma." 2003. http://www.aad.org/PressReleases/Melasma.html (15 July 2004).

American Academy of Facial Plastic and Reconstructive Surgery, Glossary (2001). Available at http://www.facial-plastic-surgery.org/patient/procedures/glossary.html (4 August 2004).

American Cancer Society. "2004 Facts and Figures." 2004. www.cancer.org (4 Nov 2004).

Associated Press. "New Research Offers Explanation of Why Smokers Look Older." *Health Central*, March 2001. http://www.HealthCentral.com.

Bank, David E., MD, with Estelle Sobel. *Beautiful Skin: Every Woman's Guide to Looking Her Best at Any Age*. Holbrook, MA: Adams Media Corporation, 2000.

Beauty and Health. "Determining Your Skin Type" (Quiz). 2004. http://www.beautynhealth.com.hk/en/analysis/skin.html (27 July 2004).

Bergfeld, Wilma, MD, FACP, with Shelagh Ryan Masline. *A Woman Doctor's Guide to Skin Care: Essential Facts and Up-to-the-minute Information on Keeping Skin Healthy at Any Age*. New York: Hyperion, 1995.

Black, Rosemary. "Skin Deep." *Vegetarian Times,* no. 293 (January 2002):28.

Bottom Line Personal, eds. *The Book of Inside Information*. Greenwich, CT: Boardroom Classics, 1995.

Boyd, Alan S., MD. *The Skin Sourcebook*. Los Angeles: Lowell House, 1998.

British Association of Dermatologists. "Sunshine and Skin Cancer." 1999. http://www.bad.org.uk (4 November 2004).

Central Practice. "Acne," 2004. http://www.centralpractice4mg.com/acne.htm (20 July 2004).

Dermatology Dictionary (2002). Available at http://www.avreskin care.com/misc/about_skincare/dermatology_dictionary.html (4 August 2004).

Dermatology Terms (2001–2004). Available at http://www.AOCD.org/skin/dermatologic_diseases/dermatology_terms.html (4 August 2004).

Dorr, Robert, PhD. "Effects of a Superpotent Melanotropic Peptide in Combination with Solar UV Radiation on Tanning of the Skin in Human Volunteers." *Archives of Dermatology* 140 (July 2004):827–835.

Draelos, Zoe Diana, MD. American Academy of Dermatology, Public Resources, 2003. "Top Ten Cosmetic Do's and Don'ts for Women with Sensitive Skin." http://www.aad.org/PressReleases/Draelos%20-%20Cosmetics.html (15 July 2004).

"Face and Skin, Makeover." *InStyleMakeover*, Fall 2004:145–148.

Gorgos, Diana, MS, BS, RN. "Eat Right, Age Less in the Sun." *Dermatology Nursing*, no. 5 (October 2002):338(1).

Haas, Elson, MD. "Staying Healthy with Nutrition." *World Health Online*, July 2001. www.worldhealth-ol.com (4 November 2004).

Health Magazine, ed. *Women's Health Confidential: 101 of Your Most Intimate Health Questions Answered*. Oxmoor House: 2001.

Hempel, Karl, MD. "The Treatment of Acne," *Health Gazette Newsletter*, February 1997. http://www.tfn.net/healthgazette (4 November 2004).

Henner, Marilu, with Laura Morton. *Total Health Makeover*. New York: Regan Books, 1998.

ICBS. "Dry Skin." Holistic-Online, 1998–2004. http://1stholistic.com/Beauty/skin/skin_dry.htm (27 July 2004).

ICBS. "Oily Skin." Holistic-Online, 1998–2004. http://1stholistic.com/Beauty/skin/skin_oily.htm (27 July 2004).

iEnhance.com. "How to Select a Qualified Dermatologist." 2004. http://www.ienhance.com/specialty/select_dermatology.asp?specialty=iedermatology (27 July 2004).

Jefferson Health System. "Scars." Frankford Hospitals. http://www.frankfordhospitals.org/healthinfo/adult/derm/scars.html (15 July 2004).

Krafert, Craig, MD. "Putting Your Best Face Forward: Treating Acne and Rosacea." Redding Dermatology Medical Group, 2001. http://www.reddingdermatology.com/acneros.htm (15 July 2004).

Leffell, David J., MD. *Total Skin: The Definitive Guide to Whole Skin Care for Life*. New York: Hyperion, 2000.

Mayell, Hillary. "Skin as Art and Anthropology." *National Geographic News*, November 13, 2002. http://news.nationalgeographic.com.

McVeigh, Gloria. "Stay Younger Longer." *Prevention* 56, no. 5 (May 2004):77.

The Methodist Hospital, *Dermatology Glossary* (2004). Available at http://www.methodisthealth.com (4 August 2004).

Mitchell, Tedd, MD. "Taking Care of Your Skin." *USA Weekend*, 9–11 July 2004.

"Mole or Melanoma?" *Consumer Reports on Health* 8, no. 11 (November 1996):130.

Narins, Rhoda S., MD, and Paul Jarrod Frank, MD. *Turn Back the Clock without Losing Time: A Complete Guide to Quick and Easy Cosmetic Rejuvination*. New York: Three Rivers Press, 2002.

Novick, Nelson Lee, MD. *Super Skin: A Leading Dermatologist's Guide to the Latest Breakthroughs in Skin Care*. New York: Crown Publishers, 1988.

The Ohio State University Medical Center. "Birthmarks." 2003. http://careconnection.osu.edu/diseasesandconditions/otherhealthtopics/Dermatology/SkinGrowths.html (27 July 2004).

The Ohio State University Medical Center. "Other Benign Skin Growths." 2003. http://careconnection.osu.edu/diseasesandconditions/otherhealthtopics/Dermatology/SkinGrowths.html (27 July 2004).

Olshansky, S. Jay, et al. "No Truth to the Fountain of Youth." Special edition, *Scientific American* 14, no. 3 (June 2004):98.

The 100 Skin Care Terms You Need to Know (2000). Available at http://www.sunandskin.com/glossary.html (4 August 2004).

Perricone, Nicholas. *The Perricone Prescription*. New York: HarperCollins, 2002.

Primedia. "Effects of Sun on the Skin: Visible Skin Changes Caused by UV Radiation." Dermatology.About.Com, 2004. http://dermatology.about.com/cs/skinanatomy/1/blsuneffect2.htm (20 July 2004).

Raichur, Pratima, with Marian Cohn. *Absolute Beauty: Radiant Skin and Inner Harmony through the Ancient Secrets of Ayurveda*. New York: Harper Collins, 1997.

Reilly, Colleen. "Antioxidants and Skin Care: Media Hype or Wonder Drug?" Vanderbilt University, Psychology Department, 27 July 2004. http://www.vanderbilt.edu/AnS/psychology/health_psychology/anoxres.htm.

Reuters Health. "Smokers Advised to Quit Before Plastic Surgery." *HealthCentral*, September 2001. http://www.healthcentral.com (4 November 2004).

"Saving Your Skin." *Harvard Health Letter* 21, no. 1 (November 1995):8(1).

Scheman, Andrew, MD. *Pocket Guide to Medications Used in Dermatology*. Palo Alto, CA: Syntex Laboratories, Inc., 1987.

Scheman, Andrew, MD, and David L. Severson. *Pocket Guide to Medications Used in Dermatology*. 5th ed. Baltimore: Williams and Wilkins, 1997.

Schoen, Linda Allen, and Paul Lazar, MD. *The Look You Like: Medical Answers to 400 Questions on Skin and Hair Care*. New York: Marcel Dekker, Inc., 1990.

"Smoking Triples Risk of Common Type of Skin Cancer." *Cancer Weekly*, 16 January 2001.

Sullivan, Colleen, et al. "The Latest Wrinkle-Fighter." *Health* 18, no. 4 (May 2004):25.

"Ten Steps to Beautiful Skin: Limit Your Alcohol Intake." *Energy Times*, March/April 1995.

Thompson Healthcare. "Dealing with Skin Problems." PDR Health, 2003. http://www.pdrhealth.com/content/rx_drugs/chapters/fgrx15.shtml (9 July 2004).

Travis, John. "Dying Before Their Time." *Science News* 166 (10 July 2004):26–28.

Warner, Jennifer. Reviewed by Brunilda Nazario, MD. "Misinformation Abounds on Anti-Aging Products." *WebMD Medical News*. 13 May 2004. http:content.health.msn.com/content/article/87/99341.htm

Warner, Jennifer. Reviewed by Brunilda Nazario, MD. WebMD Medical News, "New Drug May Help You Tan Quicker, Safer." http://content.health.msn.com/content/article/90/100874.htm (27 July 2004).

"Your Appearance." *Bottom Line* Personal, 15 July 2004:15.

INDEX

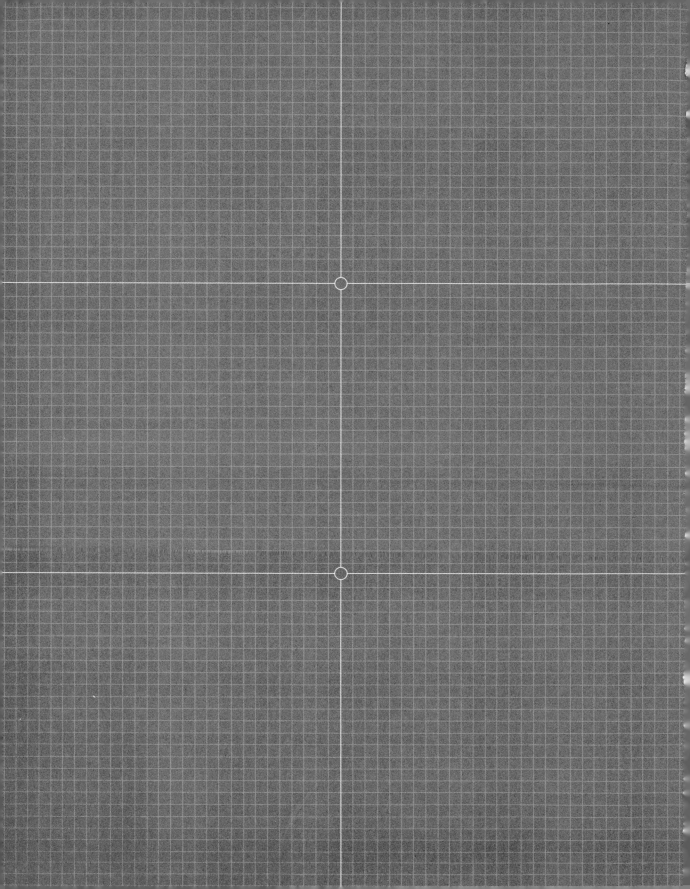